Nursing Spinal Cord Injuries

Nursing Spinal Cord Injuries

Edited by
Nalzina M. Woll CRNP, MSN

ROWMAN & ALLANHELD
PUBLISHERS

ROWMAN & ALLANHELD

Published in the United States of America in 1986
by Rowman & Allanheld, Publishers
(a division of Littlefield, Adams & Company)
81 Adams Drive, Totowa, New Jersey 07512.

Library of Congress Cataloging-in-Publication Data
Main entry under title:

Nursing spinal cord injuries.

  Bibliography: p. 151
  Includes index.
  1. Spinal cord—Wounds and injuries—Nursing.
I. Woll, Nalzina M., 1925-   . [DNLM: 1. Spinal Cord
Injuries—nursing.   WY 160 N9769]
RD594.3.N87 1986   617'.482044   85-26285
ISBN 0-8476-7380-4
ISBN 0-8476-7387-1 (pbk.)

  86 87 / 10 9 8 7 6 5 4 3 2 1
Printed in the United States of America

This book is affectionately dedicated to all the students in the Spinal Cord Injury Nurse Practitioner Program at the Veterans Administration Medical Center and California State University, Long Beach, who gave so generously of their time and effort.

Contents

Contributors

Merry Brinkley RN, BSN
Spinal Cord Injury Nurse Practitioner
Veterans Administration Medical Center
Hampton, Virginia

Mary Jane Callahan RN, BSN
Spinal Cord Injury Nurse Practitioner
Outpatient Department
Veterans Administration Medical Center
Hines, Illinois

Mary Ann Carroll RN, BSN
Spinal Cord Injury Nurse Practitioner
Veterans Administration Medical Center
Castlepoint, New York

Annie Coots RN, BSN
Spinal Cord Nurse Practitioner
Long Beach, California

June Crabtree RN, BSN
Spinal Cord Injury Nurse Practitioner
Long Beach, California

Laurene T. Dwyer RN, BSN
Clinical Nurse Specialist/Spinal Cord Injury Nurse Practitioner
Veterans Administration Medical Center
Phoenix, Arizona

Jane Egan RN, BSN
Clinical Nurse Specialist/Spinal Cord Injury Nurse Practitioner
Veterans Administration Medical Center
Indianapolis, Indiana

Karen Farrell RN, MA
Spinal Cord Injury Nurse Practitioner
Veterans Administration Medical Center
East Orange, New Jersey

Margaret Ford RN, BSN
Spinal Cord Injury Nurse Practitioner
Ranch Los Amigos Hospital
Downey, California

Mary H. Gardenhire RN, MSN
Clinical Nurse Specialist/Spinal Cord Injury Nurse Practitioner
Veterans Administration Medical Center, Lenwood Division
Augusta, Georgia

Susan Grogan RN, BSN
Spinal Cord Injury Nurse Practitioner
Mt. Rainier, Maryland

Sandra A. Harrison RN, BSN
Spinal Cord Injury Practitioner
Patient Education Coordinator
Veterans Administration Medical Center
Memphis, Tennessee

Isabelle R. Hollis ARNP, MSN
Clinical Nurse Specialist/Spinal Cord Nurse Practitioner
James A. Haley Veterans Administration Medical Center
Tampa, Florida

Deborah M. Huml RN, BSN
Clinical Nurse Administrator
Acute Spinal Cord Injury and Rehabilitation
Veterans Administration Medical Center
Hines, Illinois

Jeannette Iturrino RN, BSN
Spinal Cord Injury Nurse Practitioner
Hemodialysis
Veterans Administration Medical Center
Long Beach, California

Bonnie Johnson RN
Spinal Cord Injury Nurse Practitioner
Independent Practitioner
Long Beach, California

Alice B. McRoy RN, BSN
Spinal Cord Injury Nurse Practitioner
McQuire Veterans Administration Medical Center
Richmond, Virginia

Kathleen Morton RN, BSN
Spinal Cord Injury Nurse Practitioner
Long Beach, California

Margaret M. Murphy RNC, MSN
Spinal Cord Injury Nurse Practitioner
Director of Outpatient Clinic, Spinal Cord Injury
Rancho Los Amigos Hospital
Downey, California

Helen Pautsch RN
Spinal Cord Injury Nurse Practitioner
Rancho Los Amigos Hospital
Downey, California

Charles Pye RN, BA, BSN
Spinal Cord Injury Nurse Practitioner
Brocton/West Roxbury Veterans Administration Medical Center
West Roxbury, Massachusetts

Margaret Ann Severson RNC, FNP, BSN
Spinal Cord Injury Nurse Practitioner
Spinal Cord Clinic and In-Health Promotion Clinic
Veterans Administration Medical Center
Seattle, Washington

Jeanne Stack RN, BSN
Spinal Cord Injury Nurse Practitioner
Quincy, Ohio

Wilma Taylor CRN, BSN
Spinal Cord Injury Nurse Practitioner
Veterans Administration Medical Center
Cleveland, Ohio

Teresa Owen Tempkin RN, BSN
Spinal Cord Injury Nurse Practitioner
Nicholasville, Kentucky

William Worth RN, BSN
Spinal Cord Injury Nurse Practitioner
Daniel Freeman Medical Center
Marina del Ray, California

Preface

Literature tells us how devastating and catastrophic a spinal cord injury can be. There are an estimated 200,000 spinal cord–injured people in the United States today. Thousands more become permanently disabled every year due to damage to the brain and/or spinal cord. Suddenly, in a matter of seconds, independent people, in complete control of their lives and environment, become spinal cord injured and often entirely dependent upon others for their very existence. The most basic functions of the body may be lost. Spinal cord injuries are calamitous physically, emotionally, psychologically, socially and financially for all those who suffer them.

Descriptions of spinal cord injuries were found in ancient Egyptian tombs, but it was not until after World War II that any dramatic progress developed in caring for spinal cord–injured people. From that point on, it was recognized that there was an important need to provide quality medical and nursing care, from the moment of injury, through the critical hospitalization, and throughout the complete rehabilitation phase, until the injured person could return to the community as a useful, contributing citizen, regardless of his disability.

There are many ramifications of spinal cord injuries. Primary acute medical and nursing care is directed usually to stabilization of the injury. This book begins after the acute injury has been stabilized and is directed toward the rehabilitative aspects. These include the prevention and treatment of pressure areas, the spasticity experienced in limbs, and the common medical conditions that affect spinal cord–injured patients. This book also encompasses metabolic upsets, disturbances of the autonomic nervous system, respiratory and urinary problems, as well as disturbances of sexual functioning.

The chapters deal with the incidence, epidemiology, etiology, and pathophysiology of each problem discussed. The psychological components and the subjective and objective findings as well as the management of each disordered state are discussed. Patient and family education is critical to maintenance of quality care. Emphasis is placed on including the injured client as well as significant others in self-management. This book provides the nurse or care-giver of spinal cord patients with conceptual information on common conditions that complicate the clients' problems. It also provides injured clients and their families with information on disorders associated with their injury that may occur. It gives information on preventive measures that may be taken and on indicators that intervention is required. Being alert to these indicators during the early period promotes the seeking of medical assistance, which increases the success rate of the treatment. It is hoped that this book will promote better understanding, communication, and respect between the spinal cord injury care-givers, their clients, and significant others, which, in turn, will inevitably result in the higher quality of care.

Into the mind of every clinician who cares for a spinal cord–injured person comes the question "Are we doing all in our power to provide the most up-to-date and comprehensive care for our client?" Contributors to this book have all been trained as spinal cord injury nurse practitioners. They are dedicated to the principles of providing quality, comprehensive care to spinal cord–injured clients. The main goal of the care is to return clients to the community able to manage their lives effectively.

An expression of thanks must be given to the Long Beach Veterans Administration Medical Center, Spinal Cord Injury Service, and to the doctors who generously gave their time and knowledge to prepare the Spinal Cord Injury Nurse Practitioners. A special thank you to Dr. Stanley Gordon, Chief of Spinal Cord Injury Service, for his devotion and support in providing meaningful clinical experiences.

The editor would like to express appreciation to Dr. Margaret Koehler, professor at California State University, Long Beach, for her participation, and to Marie Carley, Associate Chief, Nursing Education, Long Beach Veterans Administration Medical Center, for her support and contribution in making the program a successful and meaningful experience.

1

Overview of Spinal Cord Injury

NALZINA M. WOLL

Spinal cord injuries have occurred since our ancestors walked upright. Primitive man fell from rocks, medieval man was thrown from his horse, and modern man sustains injuries from a car accident. Circumstances may differ, but the results are similar! The accidents result in the vertebrae being broken or dislocated and the cord being damaged, and paralysis of varying degrees ensues.

The earliest written documentation of spinal cord injury dates from the fourth century B.C. when an Egyptian physician wrote: "When examining man suffering from injury, you will find he is unaware of his hands and feet, his penis is erect, his urine escapes without him knowing it, he is flatulent and his eyes are red." He classified these injuries as "treatable diseases," "diseases I will not fight," or "diseases which cannot be treated." Sometime in the second century after Christ, a Greek physiologist distinguished different symptoms corresponding to different levels of injury. At about the same time, traction devices were being used to "straighten" the spines of injured patients.

For 1700 years, little progress was made in the treatment of spinal cord injuries. During World War II, an increase in the number of injuries occurred at about the same time as the advent of antibiotics. This, coupled with rapid transportation and improved rehabilitation techniques, resulted in great strides being made in both emergency care at the site of the accident and in expediting movement of the injured to appropriate facilities for treatment, stabilization, and rehabilitation. In the 1940s Dr. Donald Munro, often referred to as "the father of paraplegiology" and the founder of spinal cord care in 1936, emphasized that "with proper treatment, almost every patient with a spinal cord injury below the C2 to C3 level can be trained to lead a productive and rewarding life."

ETIOLOGY

It has been documented in the literature that clients who are prone to accidents resulting in spinal cord injury have a specific profile. It is an injury of the young adult, usually the aggressive male who is prone to take chances. Etiology has been classified into four categories:

1. Automobile accidents are the most common cause. Approximately 50 percent of all spinal cord injuries are due to automobile or motor-cycle accidents. High-velocity accidents tend to result in the most severe injuries.
2. Athletic or sports-related accidents account for approximately 25 percent of spinal cord injuries.
3. Gunshot and stab wounds account for approximately 15 percent of the injuries.
4. Suicide attempts, industrial, agricultural, and domestic accidents, and postoperative complications account for the remaining 10 percent of spinal cord injuries.

The normal life expectancy of American males, according to Metropolitan Life Insurance Co. tables, is 70 years. At the present time, the spinal cord–injured person who receives quality care can have the same life expectancy as the non-spinal cord–injured client. The loss of life in spinal cord injury usually occurs during the first three months of injury. Those suffering C1–C3 level injuries (see Appendix) most frequently succumb at the site of the accident. The most common cervical injuries are to C5 and C6 cervical segments, and these clients will survive with proper care.

TREATMENT

Management of acute spinal cord injury can be divided into two locations of treatment: the site of the accident and the emergency room. At the site of the accident, priority must be given to the ABCs of care: clearing the airway, and stimulating breathing and circulation. Severe hypoxia or circulatory failure can cause serious, irreversible central nervous system impairment or possible death. Loss of mobility or sensitivity (determined by pinching or touching) is sufficient reason for avoiding turning or moving the injured client. The victim must not be moved until sufficient help arrives unless his life is endangered by fire or explosion.

A most important concept is to suspect cervical injury in patients with wounds of the face, head, and shoulders and in any patient who has lost consciousness. The cardinal rule is that any head injury must be treated as a cervical spine injury until proven otherwise. Conversely, any cervical spinal cord injury must be treated as a head injury until proven otherwise. Signs and symptoms may include a dilated pupil (can be a finding in a head injury as well as a spinal injury), paralysis of the extremities, pain in head or neck, and signs of shock. Proper transportation is extremely important. The injured party must be transferred by at least four people and placed in a supine position on a firm flat stretcher or board. Preferably, a cervical collar should be applied to immobilize the neck. Sand bags may be used if a collar is not readily available. Flexion and extension of the neck must be avoided at all costs. The head and trunk must be attached to a solid, flat surface. Any objects in the injured person's pockets should be removed to prevent pressure areas. The object of treatment at the site is to prevent further injuries or complications.

Treatment in the emergency room is extremely critical. The patient must be examined before being transferred from the ambulance stretcher or spine board. Most authorities agree that the injured person must be treated with steroids, usually Decadron (dexamethasone is the generic name), within two hours of injury in order to minimize edema of the spinal cord and spinal shock. Several major concerns confront the admitting physician in the emergency room. Let's examine the presenting problems, and the proper modes of their management. The physician notes associated injuries, including life-threatening signs and symptoms.

1. He assesses *respiration and circulation* as quickly as possible and any conditions that may compromise the circulatory system. He checks:

- vital signs (TPR) and blood pressure
- color of nailbeds
- color of skin
- airway and documents air exchange
- and documents responsiveness.

If one or more of these clinical criteria is abnormal, additional emergency care is mandatory (such as clearing the airway or performing a tracheotomy). One must also distinguish between hemorrhagic shock and spinal shock. Cervical cord transections will cause mild hypotension, bradycardia, and lowered body temperature. Shock caused by hemorrhage is accompanied by tachycardia and more severe hypotension. Patients whose phrenic nerve or intercostals are involved have compromised respirations and should never receive morphine, which would further depress respiration. Patients with lower injuries may receive narcotics since respiration is seldom significantly altered. Once the client's respiration and circulatory systems have been stabilized and the head-neck body axis has been aligned by means of halter traction collar, sandbags, and/or splinting, the physician evaluates the neurological deficit.

2. The *neurological deficit* must be evaluated as soon as possible. If the injured person is conscious, any lack of feeling or inability to move

extremities is carefully determined. The patient is questioned about pain, paresthesia, bowel and bladder function, and any specific circumstances surrounding the accident. Pain is a frequent symptom at the site of the injury, and radiation of pain along the nerve roots may indicate a fracture that causes compression of the affected nerves. The first neurological exam is the most important. It serves as a basis for future examinations, and the information gleaned provides a preliminary estimation of the extent of cord involvement. Neurological exams are repeated frequently, even hourly, if necessary. The physician:

- tests the level of motor and sensory function
- notes any responsiveness in the sacral dermatomes, such as pain on touch or pressure or any muscle activity
- interprets sensory levels over anterior-superior chest (cervical apron)
- examines perianal area carefully for sensation indicating sacral sparing, which signifies an incomplete lesion
- carefully checks reflexes, including bulbocavernous and the anal wink.

3.   The physician assesses the function of the *autonomic nervous system*, which may have suffered an acute dysfunction due to spinal shock. (Spinal shock may last from a few days to six months or longer. The longer the spinal shock, the poorer the prognosis.) The physician treats spinal shock depending on the symptoms. He

- looks for a state of areflexia, hypotension, and bradycardia. Urinary output may be low, and a paralytic ileus is not uncommon. If there are no other complications, the patient will usually have a physiological diuresis around 72 hours from the time of onset of spinal shock.
- treats hypotension with vasopressors and bradycardia with a drug, usually Atropine Sulfate.
- limits fluids to prevent overload that could lead to pulmonary edema.
- prescribes a nasogastric tube until bowel sounds are established.
- monitors intake and output by indwelling catheter for a few days, then intermittent catheterizations every four to six hours.
- establishes a bowel program early with use of suppositories and/or digital stimulation.

4.   *Orthopedic problems* are evaluated after the complete neurological assessment. Skeletal alignment is mandatory to preserve neurological integrity. Cervical spine fractures are best managed by use of traction immobilization either with the halo or with tongs. The injured client should be mobilized in three weeks if possible in a wheelchair and on a tilt table. The three common types of injury are subluxation, fracture dislocation, and compression fracture.

a. Subluxation occurs when one vertebra becomes partially dislo-
    cated with no signs of fracture. Cord damage may occur that can-
    not be treated by X-ray. Treatment is immobilization by traction
    and early stabilization by fusion.
b. Fracture dislocations usually occur in regions of greatest mobility,
    between C5 or T11 and L2 (see charts in Appendix). These inju-
    ries are usually the most severe and the most harmful kind of spi-
    nal injury.
    • Cervical fracture dislocations are treated with skeletal traction
      up to 75 pounds.
    • If there is adequate spinal column alignment and minimal neu-
      rological deficit, early fusion of dislocated bones is recom-
      mended.
    • Anterior fusions are usually done if only one level is involved;
      posterior fusions are done when several cervical vertebra are
      involved.
    • Postoperative treatment includes traction for three to six weeks,
      followed by a four-post brace for three to six months.
    • Three to four months after fusion, stress films are taken to
      evaluate results.
c. Compression fractures are the most common. These usually occur
    in the vertebral body without subluxation. Commonly only one
    body is involved, and these injuries are usually considered stable
    because the posterior bony elements (laminae, facets, and pedi-
    cles) remain intact. The anterior and posterior ligaments and
    related muscles and tendons contribute to this stability. If no ins-
    tability or neurological deficit is evident, conservative treatment
    with bed rest and immobilization is usual.
d. Thoraco-lumbar injuries usually occur from direct blows or force
    from falls and are treated with bed rest for three to four weeks.
    Muscles and ligaments usually heal in two to three weeks, frac-
    tures in approximately three months.

5. Spinal cord–injured clients with impaired sensory and motor
function may have major *abdominal injuries* without symptoms. They may
have some degree of nausea and vomiting, or they may have referred pain
to the supraclavicle area. One of the first signs of impending abdominal
pathology may be the client's inability to handle alimentation properly.

• Daily measurements of abdominal circumference may help confirm
  distension.
• A flat plate (X-ray) of the abdomen should be ordered.
• Stress ulcers are common in spinal cord–injured clients. Examination of gastric and/or rectal contents for blood will assist in detecting abdominal lesions and/or early stress ulcers.

LABORATORY STUDIES

Laboratory studies and radiological examinations cannot replace the total physical examination of the injured patient. They do, however, play a vital role in verifying the diagnosis and the extent of the injury. Baseline laboratory studies should include blood typing, CBC, hematocrit, electrolytes, urea, blood sugar, blood gases, and a urinalysis. Diagnostic lumbar puncture remains controversial as is the Queckenstedt test, since they may give false-negative results even though the spinal cord may be severely compressed.

Following emergency treatment, radiological examination should be done before the injured client is moved. This should first include the standard lateral view to rule out a fracture. Then the anterior-posterior views of the appropriate spinal area should be taken.

1. Lower cervical injury should include a swimmer's view with counter-traction on arms.
2. In cranio-cervical trauma, ondontoid or open views should be taken.
3. Additional films of the skull, chest, and abdomen should be taken in serious injuries. Tomography and myelography are done if indicated.

Transfers to various departments, such as X-ray, lab, or for special procedures, should always be accomplished with extreme caution until spinal cord injury is ruled out. The various departments should be notified in advance that the spinal cord–injured client is en route to the department, and the nurse or doctor should always accompany the patient.

In summary, prompt treatment of the spinal cord–injured patient is necessary to prevent deterioration. To minimize damage, the patient must be treated within one or two hours. Damage to the cord can ascend three levels above and descend three levels below the injury. The maximum changes usually occur in four hours. Chemical methods of treatment usually include 10–15 mg dexamethasone I.V. or 4–5 mg orally every six hours for four to five days. A one-time dose of 15–20 mg Mannitol I.V. is given. Physical methods of treatment may include traction with tongs or halo, laminectomies for decompression, durotomies, myelotomies, and cord cooling (irrigation with iced saline for 16 hours). The most important concept is that the patient must be constantly monitored with repeated neurological examinations that include testing of sensation, movement, and reflexes.

2

Autonomic Anomalies

MERRY BRINKLEY, ANNIE COOTS,
KAREN FARRELL, DEBORAH HUML,
JEANETTE ITURRINO, and CHARLES PYE

An injury that completely severs the spinal cord separates the connection between the brain, or higher centers, from that part of the body below the injury. The myriad sensory inputs to the brain, or afferent information, are therefore traumatically discontinued. The transmission of the sensations of pain, touch, vibration, temperature, and position sense no longer ascend beyond the site of transection. In addition, that part of the brain which is responsible for initiating voluntary movement, the motor cortex, is functionally and anatomically isolated from all voluntary muscles below the level of the injury. The integrative ability of the two sections is also impaired.

The law of the spinal cord states that if an individual sustains an injury to the spinal cord, at the level of injury there will never be a return of reflex activity. After the spinal shock disappears, however, there will be a return of reflex activity in every segment below the level of the injury (Comarr 1977a). The incidence of traumatic spinal cord injury in the United States is approximately 33 per million population per year. This means that there are 7 or 8 thousand new cases each year for a total of about 150,000 (McCutcher 1979). It is estimated that 40,000 of these have complete paralysis and, of these, 5,000 are quadriplegic. Some degree of autonomic imbalance occurs below the level of injury in virtually all cases, with the imbalance increasing in severity as the level of the lesion ascends. A brief explanation of the normal function of the autonomic nervous system will be given before the abnormalities that result from spinal cord injuries are discussed.

The autonomic nervous system is composed of two parts, the parasympathetic nervous system (PNS) and the sympathetic nervous system (SNS). The PNS performs delicate adjustments in homeostasis or fine-tuning of the internal environment. It is supportive of baseline metabolism and restorative function; that is, it tends to be "vegetative" in nature. The SNS, on the other hand, helps protect the body against physical, chemical, and biological injuring agents with a mass discharge or "fight or flight" mechanism, and also acts cooperatively with the PNS to maintain an optimum level of functioning.

The sympathetic and parasympathetic nerves leave the brain stem, travel down the spinal cord, and leave the cord at appropriate levels to enervate particular organs and structures. A specific cord segment enervates a specific autonomic function. Some of these autonomic functions include the regulation of temperature, perspiration, heart rate, blood pressure, urination, and many other vital body processes. The hypothalamus and brain stem are the higher centers for these autonomic functions.

The autonomic control of the cardiac output and the peripheral vascular system involves a complex SNS–PNS interaction. Two important autonomic reflexes are the baroreceptor reflex and chemoreceptor reflex. Baroreceptors or pressoreceptors, which are nerve endings sensitive to stimuli of vasomotor activity, are located in the aortic arch and carotid sinuses. Elevated arterial pressure causes the vessel walls to expand which, in turn, stimulates the stretch-sensitive baroreceptors to fire. These afferent impulses pass via Hering's nerve (also called the sinus nerve), through the glossopharyngeal nerve, to the medulla. Some afferent fibers ascend via the vagus nerve. Synapses connect not only the sympathetic and parasympathetic nuclei, and efferent arcs, but also the cerebral cortex and hypothalmic nuclei, which control hormonal secretion via the pituitary gland. A reduction in arterial pressure diminishes the stimulation of the baroreceptors, which in turn activates sympathetic outflow and inhibits parasympathetic activity. As a result the vascular smooth muscles in arterioles and veins constrict while the heart rate and myocardial contractility are augmented. In addition, adrenal medullary secretion output of antidiuretic hormone (ADH), output of adrenocorticotrophic hormone (ACTH), and aldosterone are all increased. These effects act to restore arterial pressure to its previous level. Thus, the operation of the baroreceptor system normally serves to buffer the body from a variety of influences that would otherwise produce marked alterations in arterial pressure.

Chemoreceptors are cells in the walls of several vessels in the neck and thorax that are sensitive to low oxygen content, excess carbon dioxide, acidity of blood plasma, and perhaps even the temperature of the blood. The stimulation of these may increase breathing, stimulate the vasomotor center, and inhibit vagal action. Kollai (1979) described the interaction of chemoreceptors and baroreceptors as they affect the autonomic control of the heart. When chemoreceptors are stimulated, both the PNS and SNS are activated. In spite of the resulting bradycardia, the vasoconstriction leads to an elevated blood pressure. This stimulates baroreceptors, which causes reduced sympathetic discharge and a drop in blood pressure. The actions of the two divisions of the autonomic nervous system will be discussed separately.

PARASYMPATHETIC NERVOUS SYSTEM

Since the nerves of the PNS originate in both cranial and sacral areas (see S2, S3, S4 in Appendix Figure A.1), the term *parasympathetic* has become relatively synonymous with the term *craniosacral*. The cranial portion consists of four nerves—oculomotor, facial, glossopharyngeal, and vagus—also called cranial nerves three, seven, nine, and ten, respectively. The oculomotor nerve enervates the ciliary muscles of the eye and the parotid and sub-maxillary glands. The vagus nerve serves the heart, stomach, small intestine, colon, lungs, liver, pancreas, and spleen. The sacral part of the PNS consists of the pelvic nerve, or nervi erigentes, which arises at the levels of S2, S3 and S4 and enervates the distal colon, kidney, bladder, and sex organs. The vagus nerve arises in the medulla oblongata, also called the hindbrain or brainstem and, technically, the myelencephalon. The medulla, an enlarged extension of the spinal cord, is the part of the brain just above the foramen magnum and is about one inch in length. The medulla is anatomically arranged in a bilateral fashion: the columns, nuclei and nerves about to be discussed have a contralateral counterpart. The medulla is partly composed of white matter or afferent and efferent myelinated projection tracts that extend to and from both the spinal cord and higher center of the brain. In addition to the projection tracts, the medulla contains areas of unmyelinated gray matter that is organized longitudinally into loosely arranged bands or columns. The three columns that involve the vagus nerve are the general visceral efferent column, the special visceral efferent column, and the visceral afferent column. The medulla contains other columns of gray matter which, since they have not been shown to involve the vagus, will not be considered here. These columns are subdivided into neuron pools called nuclei, which are aggregates of cell bodies, axons, and dendrites. These cell bodies are called preganglionic cell bodies because the efferent signals pass from the medulla through these preganglionic nerves before reaching the ganglia located near the structures enervated. A ganglion is similar to a nucleus in that it, too, is a mass of axons, cell bodies, and dendrites.

Much of the coordination that characterizes the autonomic nervous system occurs in these nuclei and ganglia. Nervous integration can be facilitated in these structures in four ways.

1. *Convergence*, where a response is stimulated by input from more than one source.

2. *Divergence*, when one impulse branches to stimulate multiple effectors.
3. *Reverberation*, when an impulse is recircuited to cause a longer-lasting outflow.
4. *Inhibition*, when impulses synapse with systems that provide an antagonistic effect.

Each nucleus has two types of neurons: transmission neurons, also called relay neurons, and local circuit neurons. While transmission cells have long axons connecting to other nuclei, local circuit neurons have short axons connecting many nearby cells in their own neuron pool. The processing of the incoming afferent message takes place in the nucleus with the relay cells in the nucleus being stimulated by influences derived from convergence and divergence from the receptive field in the periphery (Noback and Demarest 1981).

Three of these nuclei, one in each of the columns mentioned earlier, contribute fibers that comprise the vagus nerve. The dorsal motor nucleus of the vagus nerve is located in the special visceral efferent column, and the nucleus solitarius is found in the visceral afferent column. Unlike the first two, the visceral afferent column is not considered to be composed of preganglionic fibers, because it transmits afferent impulses, or sensory information. According to Noback and Demarest (1981) these vagal afferent impulses arise in three major areas:

1. the pharynx, esophagus, stomach, intestinal tract (to the left colic flexure), larynx, bronchi and lungs, and such organs as the liver, pancreas, and their ducts
2. pressoreceptors in the aortic arch, atrium, and the ventricles of the heart and in the pulmonary tree
3. chemoreceptors in the aortic bodies and major thoracic arteries.

Stimulation of the vagus nerve results in the release of a chemical, acetylcholine, which causes a reduction in the rate and amplitude of the heartbeat. Acetylcholine is released at all parasympathetic nerve endings. The reaction that occurs depends on the kind of receptor (nicotinic or muscarinic) at the postsynaptic site, as well as the distribution of these receptors. Muscarinic receptors are much more common and found in all postganglionic neurons of the PNS, as well as in many sympathetic neurons. Nicotinic receptors are diffuse and found throughout the PNS receptive field.

In summary, impulses that initiate parasympathetic outflow can travel into the medulla from higher centers of the brain, up the spinal cord, and via the vagal afferent fibers. Parasympathetic activity is dependent on the neurotransmitter, acetylcholine.

SYMPATHETIC NERVOUS SYSTEM

The sympathetic division of the autonomic nervous system consists of the thoracic and lumbar outflow of visceral efferent fibers (see T4–T6 segment to the L2 segment in Appendix Figure A.1) and thus is often referred to as thoraco-lumbar. The main integrative units of the SNS are a chain of ganglia that nestle bilaterally and laterally against each vertebral interspace from T1 to L2. In addition, the SNS has outlying ganglia near various organs. Like the PNS, the pathways of the SNS are also composed of two nerve cells. The first efferent component consists of cell bodies in the intermediolateral horn of the gray matter of the spinal cord. Nerve fibers from these cells pass into the spinal nerves through the anterior root and then into the ganglion. Since these efferent fibers carry messages to the ganglia, they are called preganglionic. The second part of the SNS pathway is postganglionic, having cell bodies in either the sympathetic chain or in a ganglion near the target organ. Preganglionic fibers can synapse with adjacent ganglia, pass upward or downward in the chain and synapse with one of the other ganglia in the chain, or they can pass for variable distances through one of the nerves radiating outward from the chain, finally terminating in an outlying sympathetic ganglion (Guyton 1981).

The normal SNS derives some control and modulation from higher centers. Nervous connections exist between the intermediolateral horn of the spinal cord and centers in the medulla, pons, hypothalamus, amygdala, and probably higher centers. This supraspinal sympathetic input can be either excitatory or inhibitory. Pressor responses with more or less generalized signs of increased sympathetic discharge can be induced from some hypothalamic areas, while sympatho-inhibitory responses can be directed from other hypothalamic areas (Lisander, in Brooks, 1979).

Stimulation of a nerve causes a chemical to be released at the nerve endings. These substances are called neurotransmitters because they transmit an impulse across the synapse and stimulate the nerves on the other side. Norepinephrine is released by sympathetic nerve endings. Since norepinephrine is also called adrenalin, the term *adrenergic* is used to describe the distribution and effects of this neurotransmitter.

PARASYMPATHETIC HYPERREFLEXIA

Since the vagus nerve emerges from above the level of the spinal cord, the cranial portion of the PNS is still connected to higher centers. In addition, many parasympathetic reflexes remain intact because of reflexes transmitted via the visceral afferent column and via the glossopharyngeal nerve. *Parasympathetic hyperreflexia* is the term used to describe uninhibited parasympathetic outflow, sometimes referred to as a vago vagal reflex.

Respiratory periodicity influences autonomic tone. During normal inspiration, pulmonary stretch receptors reduce the tonic activity of the vagus nerve, and conversely increase vagal activity during expiration. The exact interaction of chemo-baro and pulmonary stretch receptors is not known. However, a reflex bradycardia and cardiac arrest can occur in newly injured intubated patients on a respirator. Suctioning these patients creates a hypoxia and chemoreceptor stimulation. This stimulation normally causes secondary tachycardia as a result of the hypoxic drive. Hyperventilation is impossible in respirator patients, however, so the vagus suppression of inspiration is eliminated. The resultant vago vagal reflex can cause cardiac arrest. The precipitating factors appear to be hypoxia, intubation, and trachal suctioning. To prevent vago vagal reflex, in addition to providing adequate oxygen, atropine may be administered to block the muscarine effects of the PNS, therefore blocking vagal stimulation.

TEMPERATURE CONTROL

The autonomic control of temperature is also altered in spinal cord injuries. In the normal person, a series of peripheral and deep warm and cold sensors transmits impulses to the vasomotor center. In response to cold, a decrease in cutaneous blood flow reduces the heat transfer from the inner core of the body to the shell, or skin. Conversely, in response to heat, blood flow is diverted from the body core to the shell where it can be dissipated.

Since the vasomotor center is disconnected from all vessels below the injury, the autonomic control of temperature is lost in spinal cord injury (SCI). The body temperature of SCI patients changes in the direction of the environment. Extremes of heat or cold can be dangerous. Therefore, care must be taken to clothe patients adequately in the winter and to provide appropriate heating. Body heat dissipates rapidly in the outdoors; most quadriplegics can spend only short periods of time outside without sustaining significant temperature drops. Conversely, their temperature can elevate rapidly in hot summers. Adequate ventilation or air conditioning must be provided.

PARASYMPATHETIC HYPOREFLEXIA

The sacral portion of the parasympathetic nervous system is isolated from the higher centers after spinal cord injury. The most common autonomic problem, which occurs in 95 percent of SCI patients, is urine retention as a result of sacral parasympathetic insufficiency. Normal detrusor contraction is markedly diminished or absent in SCI, which creates a response often too weak to empty the bladder. The diagnosis of such a condition may be through sympathetic hyperreflexia, by obtaining post-voiding urine residuals, or by observing bladder distension.

Kidney failure is the highest cause of death among the SCI population. The patient must be taught that this retention leads to reflux, ascending infection, and pyelonephritis. The treatment can be by percussion and crede, or by urecholine, which is given to induce micturition. An important aspect of the teaching plan is to stress that consistency is required to prevent distension. That is, the patient must not omit medications or manual methods for bladder emptying.

SYMPATHETIC HYPERREFLEXIA

A spinal cord injury alters the chemoreceptor and baroreceptor effect of the autonomic nervous system. The ability of the body to react to changes in blood volume, pressure, and chemical composition is decreased. The inability to inhibit the SNS allows the occurrence of sympathetic hyperreflexia, which, it has been estimated, may occur in as many as 83 percent of SCI patients (Erickson 1980). A noninjured person is able to temper such outflow by inhibiting the SNS from reflex centers in the hypothalamus, coupled with the antagonistic action of the PNS. In SCI, however, a noxious stimulus from below the level of injury enervates the sensory receptors, sending afferent impulses to the spinal cord and upward to the brain. The severed cord blocks the afferent impulse from traveling up the spinothalamic tract and posterior column at the point of injury. Since the autonomic reflex in the spinal cord is intact, the blocked impulses activate a sympathetic reflex. This increased sympathetic discharge causes vasoconstriction of the skin and in the viscera. Sustained vasoconstriction of the skin and in the viscera in turn causes an increase in the resistance of blood flow and results in a very high blood pressure. This leads immediately to a pounding headache, piloerection, and sweating. This anomaly is sometimes referred to as autonomic dysreflexia, but sympathetic hyperreflexia is the preferred term.

The early sign of high center involvement is bradycardia. This occurs as a result of the vagus nerve being intact. The sudden rise in blood pressure is detected by the baroreceptors in the carotid sinus and aortic arch, triggering afferent impulses to vasomotor regulatory centers in the medulla, via the vagus and glossopharyngeal nerves, and efferent impulses by the vagus and sympathetic nerves to slow the heart rate. The sympathetic block does not allow vascular dilation to occur in the visceral and peripheral vasculature, so there are no counter forces to lower the blood pressure. The patient develops flushing in the face and neck with visibly engorged vessels of the temporal and neck areas, plus nasal congestion. Complete blockage of the nasal airway may occur. The higher the lesion in the spinal cord, the more depressed is the functioning of regulatory mechanisms (Taylor 1974).

The complications of sympathetic hyperreflexia are acute myocardial failure, and retinal or intracranial hemorrhage. Thus it is essential for the individual who shows early signs and symptoms of the anomaly to receive immediate care.

Etiology

The most common cause of sympathetic hyperreflexia is a distended bladder. This is caused by a plugged, kinked, or twisted catheter, which prevents proper drainage. Severe spastic bladder, acute genitourinary infection, kidney or bladder stones, and such urologic procedures as catheterizations, irrigation, and exploratory and surgical maneuvers can also initiate sympathetic hyperreflexia.

Other stimuli that can initiate the anomaly are bowel stimulation from stool, manual examination as in bowel care, or insertion of a suppository. Even an enema may trigger an autonomic reflex. Stimulation of the skin that could initiate a reflex includes intense pressure (including tight clothing), any painful pressure sore, pinched scrotum or testicle, a severe blow, or hot or cold air. Other possible stimuli are a severe spasm, fractured limb, certain body positions, surgical procedures, and even ejaculation in men or strong uterine contractions in pregnant women.

Signs and Symptoms

The clinical manifestations of sympathetic hyperreflexia include sudden arterial hypertension as high as 300/160, a severe throbbing headache, profuse sweating with flushed skin above the level of the cord injury, piloerection, nasal stuffiness, and bradycardia. Some individuals have also experienced pericardial pressure. The high blood pressure has added significance, since the average quadriplegic patient has a blood pressure of 90/60, and some of them have even lower blood pressure when in a sitting position. The onset of the symptoms may be gradual, but more often it is rapid, developing in a matter of seconds or minutes. The symptoms vary greatly among SCI patients.

Subjective Symptoms

1. Sudden, severe throbbing or pounding headache
2. Goose pimples
3. Sweating of face, head, and other areas above the level of the SCI
4. Stuffy nose
5. Chills without fever
6. Blurred vision

Objective Symptoms

1. Extreme hypertension, 300/150 mm Hg; for some SCI patients 140/90 can be severe
2. Bradycardia, but initially the pulse may be fast-pounding and sometimes irregular
3. Flushed skin of face and neck
4. Restlessness
5. Dilated pupils
6. Diaphoresis
7. Splotchy skin

MANAGEMENT PLAN FOR SYMPATHETIC HYPERREFLEXIA

Complaints of headache by the patient with high spinal cord injury must be taken seriously, and not treated casually with aspirin. Removing the stimulus is the immediate treatment for autonomic hyperreflexia. It is important to detect signs and symptoms early because the blood pressure will remain high, placing the patient in jeopardy, until the cause is removed or until medication is given to decrease it.

DIAGNOSTIC PLAN

Immediate

1. Observe symptoms: headache with bradycardia and elevated pressure is a sure sign of sympathetic hyperreflexia.
2. Check the urinary drainage system for obstructions.
3. Check the rectum to rule out constipation and impaction.
4. Check the toes to rule out an ingrown toenail.

Delayed

The following measures should be taken if headache persists, for it has been found that sometimes the only clinical symptoms are severe headache and profuse sweating.

1. Check the urine creatinine clearance to rule out kidney disease.
2. Order SMA 12 to rule out hypertension, cardiovascular disease.
3. Order culture and sensitivity to rule out urinary tract infection.
4. Order cystourethrogram to rule out kidney and bladder stones.

THERAPEUTIC PLAN: IMMEDIATE OR ACTIVE MANAGEMENT

For high blood pressure:

1. Elevate the head of the bed or elevate the patient's head if not contraindicated. Simply elevating the head by placing the patient in a
   sitting position has been observed to significantly lower blood pressure in quadriplegic patients. A sitting blood pressure of 90/60 is not
   uncommon in these patients. The patient must be kept in a sitting
   position until reflex symptoms subside.
2. Monitor blood pressure every one to three minutes.
3. Call a physician if the blood pressure remains elevated. The blood
   pressure varies among SCI patients. Some of them may experience
   violent symptoms with a blood pressure of 140/90, while others may
   exhibit milder symptoms with 190/100. It is difficult to determine at
   what point a physician should be notified for sustained, elevated
   blood pressure.

For bladder distention or obstruction:

1. Remove the stimulus.
2. Check the urinary drainage system for obstructions.
3. If the patient is on an indwelling catheter, check to see if the tube is
   plugged or clamped.
4. If the catheter is plugged, remove it and reinsert another. With the
   new catheter inserted, drain the urine 500 cc at a time once every ten
   minutes. If draining the first 500 cc does not lower the blood pressure, drain another 500 cc immediately. The catheter should be
   clamped between drainings. The emptied bladder should be
   watched closely for severe contractions that could cause the blood
   pressure to rise again. If this happens, it may be necessary to initiate
   drug therapy.
5. If the patient is on an external catheter:
   a. External maneuvers such as Crede should not be done. Any
      increased pressure to the distended bladder may raise blood pres-
      sure even higher.
   b. Initiate micturition by tapping lightly on the external catheter, or
      by pulling the public hair, so long as the blood pressure does not
      continue to rise. Many SCI patients establish a trigger point to
      start voiding.

If the above interventions do not initiate micturition and the blood pressure remains elevated, then other possible sources of stimulation should be
investigated.

For bowel dysfunction:

1. Bowel stimulus
2. For fecal impaction or constipation, insert a tube of nupercainal
   ointment to anesthetize the rectum before attempting manual evacu-

ation. Then wait 10 to 15 minutes before the attempt is made. In any case, the rectum should be evacuated after the symptoms subside.

3. Skin stimulus.
4. Reposition the patient to relieve the pressure area and pressure on decubitus ulcers.
5. Check windows for drafts and mechanical devices that may be disturbing the ambient air.

ACTIVE MEDICAL MANAGEMENT

For blood pressure that does not respond to nursing intervention:

1. The physician will probably intervene, ordering a ganglionic blocking agent to reduce the blood pressure. Good results have been obtained using ganglionic blocking agents administered intravenously.
2. Hydralazine (Apresoline): 1.0 ml or 20 mg is given intravenously at a rate not to exceed 0.5 ml per minute.
   a. The patient may experience severe hypotension as a response to IV hydralazine. Make sure that the hypotension did not occur because the patient hyperventilated secondary to anxiety produced by experiencing autonomic dysreflexia or because of hypoglycemia secondary to not eating.
   b. Aramine bitartrate (Aramine), an antidote for hydralazine, should be readily available. If needed, 10 mg of Aramine in 500 cc of 0.9% sodium chloride is administered IV, titrating the flow rate with the blood pressure reading to elevate the blood pressure (Comarr 1977a; Taylor 1974).
   c. A low spinal anesthetic may be necessary if hydralazine fails to lower the blood pressure. Use pontocaine hydrochloride, 6 mg in 1 ml of 10% dextrose in water, given intrathecally.

PREVENTIVE NURSING MEASURES

1. Keep the patient's catheter draining well at all times.
2. When irrigating the bladder, do not use more than 30 cc of irrigating solution at a time. Be sure to get all the fluids back out.
3. Avoid stimulating the patient's skin below the level of the injury.
4. Use gloves lubricated with Nupercainal ointment for bowel care.
5. For routine catheter changes, instill 20 to 30 cc of 0.25% Pontocaine into the bladder 15 minutes beforehand.
6. Avoid stimulating the rectal-anal area.
7. To prevent hypotension:

  a. Wrap the legs with elastic bandages or apply support hose.
  b. Apply abdominal support before getting the patient up into a sitting position or from the bed to a wheelchair.

LONG-TERM MEDICAL AND PREVENTIVE MANAGEMENT

To control symptoms of autonomic dysreflexia, oral ganglionic blocking agents or alpha-adrenergic blocking agents are sometimes given.

1. One 20 mg tablet of pentolinium tartrate (generic), which is Ansolysen (trade), every six hours, plus more if necessary, to keep blood pressure between 90–120/60–80.
2. Instead of Ansolysen, 5 to 10 mg of mecamylamine hydrochloride (generic), which is Inversine (trade), three times per day may be used. Inversine is effective in controlling sweating, but possible unwanted side effects are hypotension and constipation.
3. Phenoxygenzamine (generic), which is Dibenzyline (trade), a long-acting adrenergic alpha receptor blocking agent, is used to control episodic hypertension and sweating. The dosage is adjusted to the needs of each patient, starting with 10 mg daily and increasing until the desired effect is obtained.
4. 15 mg of propantheline USP (generic), which is Probanthine (trade), every six hours, or as necessary, is used to control bladder spasm and diaphoresis.
5. Oxybutyrin (generic), which is Ditropan (trade), in the usual dosage of a 5 mg tablet two to three times a day is used to control a reflex neurogenic bladder.
6. A 25 mg tablet of ephedrine (trade or generic) given 20 minutes before getting the patient up into a wheel chair is helpful in preventing postural hypotension.
7. Other drastic measures: to be used for patients with violent symptoms in order to completely destroy the reflex function. These measures should be taken only if other management treatments have been unsuccessful in lowering blood pressure.
    a. cordectomy
    b. pelvic or pudendal nerve section
    c. posterior sacral rhizotomy
    d. subarachnoid alcohol block
    e. transurethral bladder neck surgery
8. Local anesthesia in anal, urethral, vesical and mucosa regions is necessary before any kind of urological instrumentation or manipulation is attempted with SCI patients who are highly susceptible to sympathetic hyperreflexia.

9. The important aspect of management is early recognition of the symptoms of sympathetic hyperreflexia so that appropriate action can be taken as quickly as possible.

PATIENT EDUCATION

Many complications are a threat to the SCI patient and may cause a setback in his rehabilitation at any time. Sympathetic hyperreflexia is just one of the serious complications that plague the high SCI patient.

It is the responsibility of the nurse and the physician to include in the teaching plan of SCI patients, their families, significant others, and attendants, all information about the symptoms and management of the disorder. It is also necessary to inform the patients completely about their condition, pointing out the likelihood of susceptibility to attacks of sympathetic hyperreflexia. It is especially important that all quadriplegics and high paraplegics be thoroughly informed about their condition. Many treatment facilities prepare and distribute to anyone involved in caring for an SCI patient printed instructions and guidelines for detecting and managing an attack of sympathetic hyperreflexia.

Patients who are on an external catheter must be taught to empty their bladders at regular intervals. They must learn that skipping just one scheduled emptying may be sufficient to set off a reflex response. Even if the patient finds himself at a place that is inconvenient to emptying the bladder, he must learn not to allow himself to give into this excuse for going off schedule. Patients can be taught that by careful planning they can avoid getting into trouble. Emptying the bladder just prior to entering an inconvenient place is one preventive measure. Another is to restrict oral fluid intake at such times.

ORTHOSTATIC HYPOTENSION

Orthostatic hypotension (sometimes termed sympathetic hyporeflexia) is one of the problems presenting complications in spinal cord injury patients. Orthostatic hypotension is known to occur in patients with lesions above the T4–T6 dermatome (see Appendix Figure A.1). Orthostatic hypotension can be defined as a sudden drop in blood pressure that occurs with a change of position from lying to standing. It can also occur from lying or sitting or from sitting to standing. It is more pronounced when the change is sudden rather than gradual. The arterial blood pressure falls when the patient is in an upright position because of the absence of normal vasoconstriction when blood is pooled in the portion of the body below the heart.

A failure of vasoconstriction in response to a fall in blood pressure could result from a loss of intrinsic tone in the capillaries and arterioles, or an interference with the reflexes which regulate the arterial pressure. There is evidence that the arterioles and the capillaries are functioning normally when properly stimulated, because heat applied locally caused vasoconstriction. Thus the major factor responsible for the fall in blood pressure is malfunction of the reflexes that control the level of the arterial pressure, which in turn causes malfunction of the circulatory and hormonal mechanisms of adaptation to postural change.

As has been previously discussed, the maintenance of normal vasomotor tone depends on both central and peripheral sources. Such sources include baroreceptors, chemoreceptors, somatic activity, and perhaps a supraspinal central generating mechanism. This tonic activity provides a semiconstriction of blood vessels called vasomotor tone. These partially contracted vessels can therefore dilate, or constrict, giving the capability of bidirectional response. Upon standing, the pressure in the upper body normally falls as the blood goes to the lower part of the body. With the falling pressure in the upper portion of the body, the baroreceptors are no longer stimulated by stretching. The vasomotor center in the medulla is excited and transmits sympathetic impulses downward through the cord, resulting in vasoconstriction and a return of blood pressure to normal.

With spinal cord injury, the loss of the sympathetic vasomotor tone results in blood vessels that are not continually semiconstricted, but are in a state of vasodilation. This results in a low baseline blood pressure. Since they have an interruption of the reflex arc that normally produces vasoconstriction in the upright position, they also may have a sudden drop in blood pressure with assumption of an erect position. The loss of vasomotor tone occurs not only in the peripheral circulation, but also in the abdominal visceral circulation.

It has been found that orthostatic hypotension occurs more often with spinal cord injury lesions above T5, since this is the level of the upper extent of the sympathetic outflow to the intraabdominal viscera.

SIGNS AND SYMPTOMS

The clinical manifestations of orthostatic hypotension, in addition to the drop in arterial blood pressure, include increase in heart rate, blurred vision leading to loss of vision, tingling in the hands, tremors, headache, nausea, restlessness, pallor, cold or mottled extremities, frequent yawning, and syncope. The specific signs and symptoms vary from patient to patient, but each patient usually has the same premonitory symptoms, so it is possible to learn to anticipate the loss of consciousness and alter body position to prevent its occurrence.

MANAGEMENT

The emphasis in treatment of orthostatic hypotension is on prevention. Regular, frequent changes of posture from the supine to the lateral position and elevating the head of the bed in the early stages, following transection of cord injuries about the T-5 level, provides an important stimulus for setting up vasoconstrictor responses within the body, thus restoring some vasomotor control. Assumption of upright position should always be a gradual process, with propping on two or three pillows and gradual head raising preceding an attempt to sit on the side of the bed.

The application of an abdominal binder and elastic support stockings to the lower extremities will help circulatory adaptation. Elastic stockings should be removed at least twice daily for good skin care. Encourage deep inspirations, as this activity helps with vasoconstriction. In a high cord injury, this vasoconstriction in the hands prevents or delays fainting due to postural hypotension. The use of postural exercises in bed or on a tilt-table and weight lifting can be beneficial.

Other approaches to increasing blood volume include diet and medication. In the diet area, extra sodium chloride may be added if not otherwise medically contraindicated. Ephedrine 25 mg by mouth (p.o.) may be given 20 to 30 minutes before raising the patient from a horizontal to vertical position if more conservative measures do not alleviate the problem. Hydrocortisone in low dosages has been found beneficial in some patients in recent trials.

If orthostatic hypotension occurs when the patient is in the wheelchair, the attendant should firmly grab the handle of the wheelchair, tilt the patient backward and lower him until the head and neck are nearly horizontal with the floor. This will increase the blood pressure and the blackout should cease. The patient should then be gradually raised and lowered until his blood pressure is stabilized.

Biofeedback is one of the more experimental ways of dealing with postural hypotension. With this technique the spinal cord–injured patient may learn to control his blood pressure voluntarily. A case study reports this approach with a person having a T-3 lesion. The patient was treated for eight sessions, in which he was helped to learn how to voluntarily increase his blood pressure. It was found that a person with a spinal cord lesion at T-3 level can successfully learn to increase his blood pressure voluntarily. The reliability of the effect on the blood pressure within a few minutes after being instructed to change his pressure and the consistency of the magnitudes of the changes, along with the return of the pressure to a normal level within minutes after being instructed to stop changing it, demonstrated that the resultant changes were of a voluntary nature. While the results of this study suggest the feasibility of utilizing this approach clinically, it is still very experimental, and further research is essential (Bruckner 1977).

Teaching the spinal cord–injured patient with orthostatic hypotension is an integral part of good nursing care. The significant others and caretaker as well as the patient need to be included in the education program. The patient with orthostatic hypotension ideally should be taught the basic knowledge of the disease process and the principles regarding treatment. It is essential that the patient understand the need not to arise suddenly after being recumbent. He should learn to first exercise his legs while at rest, then sit on the side of the bed and resume exercising his legs before attempting to arise. If he becomes lightheaded or dizzy, he should return to the recumbent position. A patient is encouraged to have the head of his bed elevated 8 to 12 inches. He is taught the reason for the elastic stocking and abdominal binder and their proper application. Also as a safety feature, the patient is taught the value of seat belts in the wheel chair or automobile to eliminate further injury due to blackouts. The patient is also taught the action use, dosage, and side effects of ephedrine. After the patient is given the necessary knowledge, he should be given the opportunity to verbalize his understanding of it.

SPINAL SHOCK

Spinal shock refers to that state of diminished excitability or altered reflex activity of the spinal cord that exists for a time period ranging from several days to six or eight weeks after injury to the spinal cord has been sustained. The muscles enervated by the cord segments situated below the level of the lesion are completely paralyzed and flaccid. Muscle tone is lost and the reflex arc is abolished. If the reflex activity does not return, it is probably due to degeneration of the spinal cord secondary to vascular thrombosis following the injury (Comarr 1977a).

There is not complete agreement in the literature about the time of onset of spinal shock. Hardy and Elson (1976) believe there is a delay in the onset of spinal shock in some patients. They believe that some reflexes, such as the cremasteric reflex, the ankle tendon reflex, the bulbocavernous reflex, and the plantar responses may be present shortly after the injury but disappear in the following hours. This is suggestive of a spread of disturbance within the spinal medulla accompanied by an alteration in the neurological state. The sacral reflexes frequently show a delayed response and commonly disappear in a day or two. It has even been shown that the anal sphincter response may not disappear at all in some injuries. It is thought that these reflexes function until the remaining electrical charge in the spinal cord is finally dissipated. The alterations in activity show much variation in pattern, and there may be all levels of variation, from a state of exaggerated reflex activity to a profound depression of all reflexes. There are rare occasions when immediately following an injury a total paralysis of limbs occurs. This, though, is accompanied by an increase in reflex activity, muscle tone, and withdrawal responses to skin stimulation, with or without skin sensation in the corresponding segments. Whenever reflexes are found to be intact, it is important to test for preservation of voluntary motor and sensory activity referable to the same spinal segments.

Another explanation of the variation in the onset of shock deals with the oxygen levels within the spinal cord. Exaggerated reflex activity can be explained by a progressive oxygen debt (Hardy and Rossier 1975). Variation may be asymmetrical, and both increased activity and the depression of the activity may be present in the same case, at the same time, although in different limbs. Reflex asymmetry is usually of much less diagnostic value than are motor and sensory deficits during the acute stage of spinal cord injury. Bear in mind that the entire neurological state should be assessed as a whole. It is generally agreed that the direction of the reflex depression is from proximal to caudal; that is, that the reflex depression is more severe and of longer duration in the segments of the isolated cord situated more proximal to the transection. The distal segments will follow later. As an example, in complete transverse lesions of the cervical cord, the arm and the finger reflexes, as well as the abdominal reflexes, are abolished immediately. At the same time, the reflexes of the distal parts of the paralyzed leg, such as the ankle jerks, and in particular, reflex responses to plantar stimulation, as well as the bulbocavernous and anal reflexes, may be present or disappear only after some latent period. Guttmann (1976) sees this as proof of the dysbalance of the afferents and efferents at various levels of the spinal cord.

The plantar reflex may be permanently lost due to a conus medullaris or a cauda equina injury. These reflexes, also referred to as the Babinski reflex, are usually initially absent. It is not considered to be a reliable sign of the presence or severity of a spinal cord injury. It is felt that the only case in which the plantar response is of much practical value following an acute spinal cord injury is when an unequivocal Babinski's sign occurs in the absence of demonstrable motor or sensory deficits. Patients such as these with presumably "minimal" corticospinal tract injury merit close observation to keep on top of their neurological state.

The level of a segmental lesion in the dorsal portion of the spinal cord can sometimes be identified by the loss of the lower abdominal reflexes and the preservation of the upper ones. Even more useful is the fact that the abdominal reflexes are unilaterally diminished in amplitude or lost, or may simply fatigue rapidly on repetitive stimulation, where there is a lesion of the pyramidal tract on the same side of the body (Chused 1976).

In the cases where a diversity of reflex responses are found in the areas enervated by the same segment of the spinal cord, it is felt that these must be regarded as only partial cord transections. These will more often than not show signs of incompleteness such as the sparing of sensation in parts of the paralyzed area and in particular the sacral segments. These features lead you to believe that there is an impairment in conduction as opposed to the total loss at any given level (Hardy and Rossier 1975).

The cardiovascular system also responds to spinal shock. In most cases the blood pressure will temporarily decrease because the tonic vasomotor impulses descending from the medulla cannot pass to the thoracolumbar cord to enervate the sympathetic cells whose vasoconstriction fibers leave the cord through the anterior roots of T-1 to L-2. The decrease in blood pressure is greater in cervical lesions and less influential as the transection approaches the upper lumbar level. Later the blood pressure increases due to an independent resumption of the activity of the spinal sympathetic cells and the contraction of the smooth muscles of the blood vessels. Due to the initial decrease in the blood pressure, as well as the impaired venous circulation due to the loss of voluntary muscle contraction, the affected limbs are cold and cyanotic. This can generally be corrected with an increase in blood volume. This should be tried before utilizing medications that may have other adverse effects. There is also an absence of sweating below the level of the lesion. Along with hypotension you will note bradycardia initially. Depending on the type of lesion, as the other types of shock appear, this may change to tachycardia.

Guttmann (1976) has three theories to explain spinal shock. The first is the loss of facilitation from descending tracts. The second is the persisting inhibition from below acting upon the extensor reflexes, and the third is the axonal degeneration of the interneurons. As a general rule of thumb, the reflex arc, an important reflex mechanism, will initially be impaired due to the trauma and the injury itself. The function of the nervous system is intimately concerned with the patient's adaptation and adjustment to an everchanging environment. The reflex arc, which is the functional unit of nervous activity, begins with the receptor, a mechanism specially designed to receive stimuli. These are conveyed by sensory fibers (the afferent path) to a reflex center where they undergo elaboration and distribution. They then reach the motor fibers (the efferent path) that carry "executive" impulses to effector organs such as muscles or glands.

When dealing with spinal cord–injured patients it is important to remember that the symptoms of pain will not be felt below the level of the lesion, especially during spinal shock. This is particularly significant with the acute cord-injured patient when the emphasis is placed on treating the neurological deficit. One must not lose sight of the possibility of abdominal injuries. These will be especially difficult to diagnose due to the lack of sensation.

Although some persons believe spinal shock can persist for six months, most sources indicate it will diminish in six to eight weeks. Septic conditions resulting from pressure sores, which patients in spinal shock are extremely susceptible to, and infections of the urinary tract play an essential part in delaying the reflex automatism of the spinal cord. Neurological exams done during spinal shock at frequent intervals by the same examiners are of the utmost importance in determining the intensity, duration and site of spinal shock as well as evaluating the intricacy and variability of reflex return. Therefore the need for accurate records cannot be overstressed. If neurological recovery is to occur, signs of recovery will appear fairly early, and the persistence of decreased reflex activity speaks for the existence of a physiological, if not a complete, anatomical lesion. The appearance of the Babinski sign in the first few days is viewed as a welcome sign indicating an incomplete lesion. Once spinal shock subsides and the synaptic relays are released from the resistance imposed upon them, afferent impulses arising from peripheral stations of the nervous system in skin, tendons, muscles, ligaments, joints, and viscera begin to elicit their excitatory influence on the neural elements within the isolated cord (Guttmann 1976). Reflex perianal muscle contractions usually appear before the deep tendon reflexes. The body begins to perspire again. Once spinal shock has subsided an accurate assessment of the injury can be made.

ASSOCIATED SYNDROMES

Several syndromes are associated with spinal cord injuries: the Brown-Sequard Syndrome, the Acute Spinal Cord Syndrome, and an Acute Central Cord Syndrome. The Brown-Sequard Syndrome, seen in injuries where there is a hemisection of the spinal cord, is manifested by a loss of tactile discrimination, impaired touch perception and the loss of body position and joint sense on the same side of the body as that on which the cord has been divided. These sensory faculties are impaired on the trunk up to the dermatome of the cord segment at which the lesion is present. There are also signs of pyramidal tract dysfunction on the same side. Some of these signs are an increase in deep reflexes, the Babinski toe sign, diminution or absence of the abdominal reflexes, and spasticity and defective or lost voluntary motor control on the same side. On the opposite side of the body there is a loss of pain and temperature sensation. The sensory level for this modality is a few segments lower in view of the fact that pain fibers ascend in the posterior for a few segments before crossing to the spinothalamic tract on the opposite side. Functionally, the limb with the most power has the poorest sensation, and vice versa.

In an Acute Anterior Spinal Cord Syndrome a majority of the damage is located in the anterior aspect of the cord. The injury may be caused by a forward dislocation or subluxation, or compression by posterior protrusion of a vertebral body or disc. It might also be caused by a "tear drop" fracture. One will usually find complete motor paralysis indicative of damage in the corticospinal tracts, below the level of the lesion. Damage to the spinothalamic tract will reveal a loss of pain, temperature, and touch sensation. There will be preservation of light touch, proprioception, and position. These are mainly controlled by the posterior columns.

An Acute Central Cord Syndrome may possibly be caused by a hyperextension injury that results in damage of the central portion of the cord. This is most common in older men, and usually there is no bone damage. The damage to the cord is greater in the more centrally located cervical tracts supplying the upper extremities than in the peripherally-lying lumbar and sacral segments that supply the legs and bladder. The arm paralysis may be of the lower motor neuron type because the anterior horn cells that supply the cervical segments lie centrally in the gray matter.

3

Bladder and Bowel Dysfunction

LAURENE DWYER

Some of the greatest challenges facing health professionals who are interested in preserving the quality and length of life of spinal cord–injured clients are bladder and bowel dysfunctions. It becomes apparent immediately following SCI that the goals of prevention and management of bladder and bowel problems are of the utmost importance once the life-threatening problems are under control.

Since World War II, vast amounts of information have been learned about the central nervous system's control of bladder and bowel functions. There is a much better understanding today of bladder and bowel problems in SCI as well as the diseases of the nervous system. This has resulted in more comprehensive and improved management and treatment, and a decrease in the morbidity and mortality rates. Bladder and bowel dysfunction can create intolerable discomfort and embarrassment and may also result in other serious physiological problems as well as recurring urinary tract infections. These in turn often promote development of decubitus ulcers that may lead to debility and early death. Changes in urinary and bowel functions are sometimes subtle. The client may be unaware of what has occured or is occurring following his injury.

NEUROPHYSIOLOGY AND PATHOPHYSIOLOGY OF THE NEUROGENIC BLADDER AND BOWEL

There is no single classification of the neurogenic bladder and bowel. However, attempts at classification are now based on neurological principles rather than on results of nonphysiologic procedures (Comarr 1979).

The uninhibited neurogenic bladder and bowel result from interruption of pathways from the frontal cortex to the pontomesencephalic reticular formation. With this type of bladder, the client has uninhibited contractions. Voiding occurs early, bladder and bowel capacity is significantly reduced, and residual urine or stool is absent. An example would be an "infant bladder or bowel."

The reflex neurogenic bladder and/or bowel occurs when the injury is above the conus medularis. The lesion interrupts the ascending sensory and the descending motor tracts. There is no voluntary micturation, and a higher volume of residual urine is present due to the spasticity of the external sphincter muscle. Uninhibited contractions are present. The reflex neurogenic bladder is not under the control of the brain. This type of bladder or bowel is frequently referred to as an *upper motor neuron bladder* or *spastic bowel*.

The autonomic neurogenic bladder, also referred to as *lower motor neuron bladder*, occurs when the injury is below the conus medularis. The bladder is completely flaccid and volition is absent. There is increased urinary retention and the client never feels any pressure. The bowel with this injury is referred to as a *flaccid bowel*. The *sensory neurogenic bladder* results when posterior roots are cut or destroyed. In this type of bladder, the client can empty the bladder voluntarily but cannot tell when the bladder is full. In the motor paralytic bladder, sensation is present but motor is absent. The client cannot initiate micturation but can feel the full bladder. This results in high residual urines.

Spinal shock always produces an autonomic, flaccid bladder. No motor or sensory activities are present until spinal shock subsides. Management of complications arising from the various neurogenic bladders and bowels are an immediate priority. One of the most common problems seen in the SCI client today is vesiculo-ureteral reflux (VUR). Vesiculo-ureteral reflux is a condition where urine in the bladder flows back into the ureters and eventually backs up into the kidney parenchyma itself. This causes urinary tract infections and eventually results in acute or chronic pyelonephritis (Smith 1975). In most patients the valve that prevents backflow located at the uretero-vesicular junction is incompetent. The uretero-vesicular (UV) junction has the physiological value that permits urine to empty into the bladder by ureter peristalsis while preventing a reflux or backing up into the ureter. There are three components of the physiological value:

1. There are bundles of detrusor muscle fibers where the ureter passes through the wall into the bladder. The ureters are compressed during the voiding process when the bladder muscle contracts.
2. Within the bladder wall and at the point where the ureter passes into the bladder, there is an increase in elastic tissue within the ureters.
3. There is a Waldeyer's (named after an anatomist in Berlin, Dr. Wilhelm Von Waldeyer) sheath or a protective surrounding structure or body along the outer longitudinal muscle layer, which consists of detrusor fibers. Thus, when the bladder contracts during voiding, the Waldeyer's sheath prevents reflux by kinking the lower end of the ureters against the bladder wall.

The oblique course of the ureter through the bladder wall and under the mucosal flap is the valvular mechanism to prevent reflux. The firm attachment of the ureter within the trigone area helps provide fixation during bladder filling and micturation and is another mechanism to prevent vesiculo-ureteral reflux (Pearman 1973).

Many authors agree (Cook and King 1979; Guttmann 1976; Pearman and England 1973; Smith 1975) that chronic infection of the neurogenic bladder is associated with VUR and, consequently, renal disease. There is some debate, however, as to which is cause and which is effect. Fellows and Silver (1976) reported on some researchers who found that when infection is treated, reflux ceases. More often, though, reflux persists and infection is difficult to eradicate in the neurogenic bladder. Guttmann (1963) concluded that "infection of the bladder plays a very important etiological role in the development of vesiculo-ureteral reflux in causing impairment or destruction of the elasticity and valve-like action of the ureteric orifices, as a result of ureteritis and peri-ureteritis following bladder infection" (p. 185). Reflux has been produced experimentally by injecting saline into the tissues surrounding the intravesical ureter, thus mimicking the inflammation of the mucosa and submucosa that is associated with cystitis. Reflux has also been induced by placing foreign bodies in the bladder or renal pelvis in order to promote infection and edema of the UV junction (Cook and King 1979).

Conversely, reflux contributes to the occurrence of urinary infection because it provides a reservoir of residual urine, but more commonly when the UV junction is only marginally competent (Cook and King 1979). Obstruction at either the bladder neck or external sphincter level has also been deemed a probable contributing cause of VUR. The tight, spastic sphincter is believed to cause a large residual volume to accumulate in the bladder, increasing the intravesical pressure and eventually causing weakness and hypertrophy of the trigone musculature at the UV junction. Saccules or diverticuli develop at the weak points and result in a shortening of the intravesical segment of the ureter, allowing reflux to occur (Smith 1975). Cystitis, which leads to vesical wall edema, may also lead to VUR in the neurogenic bladder. The edema seems to affect the trigone and intravesical ureter and may impair valvular function. Once the infection is eradicated, however, cystography usually reveals no reflux. Studies on ureteric peristalsis and how VUR affect it have shown that where reflux was present, peristaltic activity was markedly depressed or completely absent, and free reflux occurred (Scott 1963).

INCIDENCE

In the neurologically normal population, the incidence of VUR is about 50 percent in children with urinary tract infection (UTI) and only 8 percent in adults with bacteriuria. This discrepancy can be explained by the fact that the female child usually has pyelonephritis, whereas the adult female usually has cystitis only (Smith 1975). According to Cook and King (1979), the incidence of reflux in people without urological symptoms is quite low. It varies from 0 percent to 2 percent in reported series, including premature infants and adults of both sexes. It has been noted in 13 percent of adult males with objective bladder outlet obstruction. Because the procedures used to diagnose VUR are either radiographic for short periods of time or involve nonphysiologic filling of the bladder, the true incidence of VUR remains unknown. It is apparent that reflux can be intermittent, unilateral, or bilateral.

Nearly all authors on the subject agree that there is an increased incidence of VUR in individuals of any age with congenital or acquired neurogenic bladder (Cook and King 1979; Guttmann 1976; Pearman and England 1973; Smith 1975). Although there is evidence in animals that interference with either the sympathetic or parasympathetic enervation of the trigone and distal ureter can contribute to reflux, clinically a combination of factors seems to be apparent in these persons (Cook and King 1979). Trabeculation and diverticulum formation secondary to increased intravesical pressure can make and usually results in an incompetent UV junction. The incomplete bladder emptying that is usually associated with neurogenic bladder predisposes the patient to chronic urinary tract infection and the development of bladder calculi, conditions that promote edema and inflammation of the UV junction and may interfere with its function, thus permitting reflux (Cook and King 1979; Pearman and England 1973).

The SCI literature has extensively discussed the problem of VUR in the past 25 years. The incidence is hard to pinpoint because of inconsistent follow-up after discharge from an SCI center. Several studies, however, have attempted to give some idea as to its frequency. Damanski (1968) found in his study that about 25 percent of paraplegics developed VUR. In his classic review of the problem, Hutch (1952) found that saccules were noted at the UV junction on an intravenous urogram in 60 of 94 SCI patients with reflux. Cystocopies were done on 30 of the 60 patients and 15 had a definite saccule at the UV junction. He found that the saccule may involve the detrusor muscle, which normally lies under the intravesical and intramural ureter, and weakens or destroys this muscle. When this happens, VUR often occurs because there is no longer any firm muscle for the ureter to be compressed against as the intravesical pressure rises. His operation to attempt to correct the condition will be discussed later. Fellows and Silver (1976) conducted a retrospective survey of SCI patients treated at Stoke Mandville in England from 1944 to 1963. The 39 patients who were included in the survey were followed to assess the long-term effects of reflux. Fellows and Silver found that reflux occurred with lesions at all levels of the spinal cord, when the lesion was both complete and incomplete. In 17 of the patients, renal damage resulted. In 32 of the patients, the initial intravenous urogram was entirely normal, and in 4 there was dilatation of the lower ureter.

It is frequently stated in the literature that long-standing catheter drainage (urethral or suprapubic) contributes not only to urinary infection, but to the contracture of the bladder, thus predisposing to diverticulum formation and trabeculation. VUR in SCI patients may be transient or permanent. It occurs unilaterally and bilaterally, though more often the former. It may change from one side to another in the course of alterations of bladder dysfunction. Reflux canals develop in the early months after injury in the presence of bladder dysfunction as a result of ascending infection of the UV junction and the ureter itself (Guttmann 1976). Treatment of VUR is still a matter of discussion. Tarabulcy, Morales, and Sullivan (1972) evaluated several forms of management of reflux in paraplegics. They found that of various treatment methods (scheduled voiding every two to three hours, continuous bladder drainage, transurethral resection of vesical neck, anti-reflux operation, and ileal conduit), scheduled voiding had the best success-to-failure ratio and ileal conduit the worst.

Hutch (1952) described his operative method of reimplanting the ureter after correcting saccule formation at the UV junction. Several adaptations of this surgery have been performed since 1952 with varying rates of success. In general, most agree that plastic repair of the UV junction should be approached with caution.

If urinary tract infection and outlet obstruction of the bladder can be eliminated or greatly reduced in the initial management of the neurogenic bladder, the chance of VUR can be minimized. Most urinary tract infections begin at the bladder level as cystitis, the organisms gaining entrance to the bladder via the urethra. Lapides (1974) states that frequently bacteria can be introduced into the urinary tract via the blood and lymphatic systems as well. The most common organism responsible for urinary tract infections is Escherichia coli. Other organisms that may cause infection are Proteus Vulgaris, Pseudomonis, Klebsiella, Staphylococcus aureus, and Streptococcus faecalis. Once the infecting organism has gained entry into the bladder, it must be able to survive the bladder's normal defense mechanisms. These mechanisms are twofold. The first stage is a process of dilution and mechanical washout of bacteria. Three factors are important: complete emptying of bladder; rate of urine flowing from kidneys through ureters and into the bladder; and frequency of voiding. Most bacteria are evacuated by this action. The second stage of this mechanism takes place in the bladder mucosa. Bacteria that come in direct contact with the bladder mucosa are destroyed by phagocytic and antibacterial action. The exact nature of this action remains unclear.

In the spinal cord–injured person, interference may occur in either or both of these mechanisms. The bladder may fail to empty completely or frequently enough (due to loss of appropriate enervation or obstruction). The resulting residual urine will contain a sufficient number of bacteria to negate the normal dilution effect. The remaining bacteria multiply in geometric proportions so that their numbers will double every 20 to 30 minutes (Ott and Rossier 1971). Loss of tissue integrity within the bladder may occur due to over-distention, instrumentation, or the use of an indwelling catheter. This can result in deactivation of the bladder wall defense. Impaired circulation to the bladder decreases the nutrients required to repair the damage to the bladder wall. Decreased circulation also leads to diminished antibacterial elements available for combating the infecting agent (Lapides 1974).

Comarr states that over-distention of the bladder due to uretheral obstruction or bladder dyssynergia is another causative factor in infection. This leads to changes in the bladder wall such as hypertrophy and hyperplasia. This is manifest by trebeculation of the bladder wall, which could lead to the formation of diverticula. Within these pockets, urine will be collected and held, thus permitting bacteria to multiply. In the presence of over-distention the danger of hydronephrosis or reflux must be considered. Reflux in the presence of increased intravesical pressure and urinary infection will lead to infection of the upper urinary tract.

Stone formation is another factor to be considered in urinary infection. Stones are developed by 10–15 percent of patients with bladder dysfunction (Harrison, Gittes, and Perlmutter 1979). The presence of urinary infection can lead to the development of struvite stones or "stones of infection" and vice versa. Urea-splitting organisms such as Proteus mirabilus in conjunction with an elevated urine pH are always associated with struvite stones. These calculi consist of magnesium, ammonium, calcium and phosphate. They form a nucleus around a foreign body such as suture material or a foley catheter, or they may reach a high enough density to create their own nucleus. These stones not only form in the presence of infected urine, but they can contain active bacteria within them, which can produce urinary infection (Harrison, Gittes, and Perlmutter 1979).

PSYCHOLOGICAL COMPONENTS

Spinal cord–injured clients must change their whole lifestyle in an attempt to adapt to their catastrophic injury. Adjusting to life in a wheelchair and all of its complications becomes a daily struggle. They must work through their loss of body function and impaired body image. They usually pass through the stages of shock, denial, depression, and anger before coming to some semblance of adjustment. A client who has not adjusted and adapted to the lifestyle in a wheelchair may act out by abusing his body in a variety of ways. One way may involve not following through on care of the bladder, poor fluid intake, not emptying the bladder as scheduled, poor hygiene, poor care of the foley or catheterization equipment, and inadequate follow-up of the urinary tract after injury. Any of these could result in chronic UTI which, as previously mentioned, is a primary factor in the development of VUR. The loss of control over bodily function is another insult to the already damaged body image. The patient experiences a loss of personal privacy in that a region of his anatomy, which has always been private, has become a center of attention due to his infection. A patient with a high-level injury must depend on nursing personnel or husband, wife, mother, father or significant other for the maintenance of urinary drainage.

Another aspect of concern for the individual is the possible transmission of the urinary infection to a sexual partner during intercourse. This is especially true in individuals with chronic urinary infections. This may create another stumbling block to successful post-injury sexual adjustment. Many times the individual may fear the need for surgical intervention to prevent urinary infection or to treat the post-infection damage. This individual is apprehensive about having a sphincterotomy to ensure adequate drainage of his bladder, as it may cause the loss of erectile capability. Other forms of surgery may be disfiguring (as in cutaneous vesicostomy) or may present more obstacles to independence.

Through patient education and observation of other spinal cord–injured persons, the individual becomes aware of the seriousness of urinary infections and of the complications that may arise from them.

ASSESSMENT INDICATORS OF URINARY AND BOWEL DYSFUNCTION

SUBJECTIVE DATA

Subjective data include history of preinjury urinary and bowel function, including fluid intake, exercise, diet, urinary and bowel habits, as well as personal hygiene and habits. Frequently heard comments on present function include:

"I can't empty my bladder completely."
"I have a chronic bladder infection. It never goes away."
"My kidneys hurt all the time."
"My urine residuals are always over 150 cc."

"I haven't felt well for months."
"I'm leaking around my catheter."
"My urine smells bad."
"I have chills and fever frequently."
"I have increased spasms in my abdomen and legs."
"I have diarrhea all the time."
"I'm constipated all the time."
"I have involuntary stools in spite of my bowel training program."

Rarely do spinal cord–injured patients complain of typical symptoms such as urgency, pain and burning on urination, or on having a bowel movement.

The client with a high-level lesion (T-6 or higher) may complain of symptoms of autonomic dysreflexia (see Chapter 2).

OBJECTIVE DATA

In urinary tract infections, a physical examination is of limited value (Stefan 1978). Indicators of urinary problems include:

1. Concentrated urine with large amounts of mucus-shreds, casts, egg shell calculi, and/or blood.
2. Bladder trabeculations and bladder spasms (may or may not feel tenderness when abdomen is palpated).
3. VUR documented on Cystourethrogram.
4. Elevation of temperature, pulse, and blood pressure.

Indicators of bowel problems are:

1. Dark, tarry stools or bright red blood in stools.
2. Watery stools and/or an increased amount of mucus.
3. Symptoms of bowel obstruction with small involuntary stools.

MANAGEMENT

DIAGNOSTIC PLAN

1. A complete history and physical exam, including chest X-ray and abdomen X-ray, if indications of bowel dysfunction are present.
2. A complete neurological examination (see Chapter 8).
3. A complete urological examination with diagnostic studies including:
   a. Urinalysis with culture and sensitivity.
   b. Complete blood count with differential.
   c. Electrolyte and metabolic panels (SMA 6 and 12 or equivalent).
   d. Measurement of residual urine.

    e. Cystourethrogram (CUG).

    f. Intravenous urogram or Renal Scan (if allergic to dye).

    g. Cystocopy if indicated.

    h. Ultrasound if cyst or tumor is suspected.

4. A complete GI examination for bowel dysfunction, including Upper GI Series (UGI) and a Barium (Ba) enema.

THERAPEUTIC PLAN FOR BLADDER DYSFUNCTION

1. If VUR is documented on X-ray and if urine residuals are consistently over 150 cc, refer to urologist for possible sphincterotomy or a transurethral resection of the bladder neck.
2. Attempt to relieve bladder distention by increasing intermittent catheterization until GU workup can be accomplished and GU status can be evaluated.
3. Treat urinary tract infections with appropriate measures.

    a. Use of appropriate antibiotic based on culture report.

    b. Antipyretics for febrile clients every four hours as needed.

    c. Increase fluid intake to a least three liters daily.

    d. Bedrest if symptoms are severe.

4. Chronic asymptomatic urinary tract infections should not be treated with antibiotics, since this predisposes to the development of resistant bacteria (Harrison, Gittes, and Perlmutter 1979).
5. Medications such as Banthine or Ditropan may be ordered to control uninhibited contractions of the bladder, or medications such as Dibenzyline to relax the bladder neck.

PATIENT EDUCATION

It is essential that SCI clients and their families understand what they are being treated for and what the treatment consists of.

1. Discuss preventative factors such as adequate fluid intake, good personal hygiene, activity, no bubble baths, cotton underwear, and so forth.
2. Review with the clients and their families how to avoid and treat infections and reflux in the neurogenic bladder, such as increased fluid intake and avoidance of juices that contain urea splitting acids.
3. Teach the clients and their families the correct procedure of intermittent catheterizations, making certain they understand why it is essential to try to eliminated residual urine in the bladder. If an indwelling catheter is essential, teach correct care of catheter and perineal hygiene.

4. Discuss most common bowel and bladder problems
   a. Review all prescribed medications and side effects.
   b. Take *all* antibiotics prescribed even if patient feels well.
   c. An adequate diet, increased fluids, and appropriate activity and exercise are vital.
   d. Notify physician if condition worsens.
   e. Stress the importance of follow-up evaluations and annual preventative check-ups.

4

Hemodialysis in End Stage Renal Disease

SANDRA A. HARRISON

INTRODUCTION

In spite of the tremendous advances made toward diagnosing, treating, and preventing complications in the spinal cord injury (SCI) patient, renal disease continues to be the major threat to this patient population (Mirahmadi and Winer 1977). The phenomenon of a neurogenic bladder and the invasiveness of catheters and certain diagnostic techniques predispose the SCI patient to urinary tract infections (Stamey 1980:20). Along with other clinical findings, end stage renal disease is diagnosed when the creatinine clearance falls below 10 ml per minute and the blood urea nitrogen (BUN) exceeds 80 mg/dl. Due to the chronic presence of bacteria in the urine, the SCI patient with end stage renal disease does not have the alternative of a kidney transplant. Hemodialysis is the only other alternative to death for this patient.

This chapter defines and discusses several important factors involved with hemodialysis of the SCI patient. Much of the information presented in this chapter has been obtained from the SCI Hemodialysis Unit at the Veterans Administration Medical Center in Long Beach, California (LBVAMC). The various types of equipment as well as peritoneal dialysis are beyond the scope of this chapter and will not be discussed.

INCIDENCE AND EPIDEMIOLOGY

The exact incidence of end stage renal disease in SCI is unknown, but it is estimated that up to 75 percent of the deaths in SCI are due to renal failure. The major contributing factors in the development of renal failure in SCI are chronic pyelonephritis, calculus disease, amyloidosis, and hypertension (Mirahmadi and Winer 1977; Tribe and Silver 1969). The presence of chronic bacteruria may predispose this population to any of the factors leading to renal disease. Approximately 80 percent of SCI patients have bacteria in their urine (Stamey 1980:547). Chronic, indwelling foley catheters are widely used to drain the neurogenic bladder. It has been found that 98 percent of patients with an indwelling catheter for more than four days will develop bacteremia despite the administration of prophylactic antibiotics (Yashon 1979:304). Intermittent catheterizations, i.e., every four to six hours around the clock, have demonstrated a decrease in the incidence of urinary tract infections. This is thought to be due to the zero residual volumes from the frequent bladder drainage (Merritt 1981).

PATHOPHYSIOLOGY

In order to understand the pathophysiology of end stage renal disease, the normal functions of the kidney must be understood. The kidney provides four main functions: (1) filtration, (2) excretion, (3) reabsorption, (4) secretion (Beland and Passos 1975:477). Assuming normal kidney function, a minimum of 500 ccs of fluid per day must be excreted as urine to prevent an accumulation of metabolic wastes (Harvey and Johns 1980:100). The kidney excretes excess water and products of metabolism, particularly products of protein catabolism (urea, creatinine, uric acid). It also regulates the constancy of the internal environment by maintaining the volume of water, the electrolytes, osmolality, and the hydrogen ion concentration of the extracellular fluid (Beland and Passos 1975:477).

Erythropoietin is a hormone secreted from the kidney that influences red blood cell formation in bone marrow (Papper 1971:81). The kidney also produces the enzyme renin. Renin production will increase in the presence of decreased renal perfusion. This increase in renin stimulates the release of aldosterone from the adrenalcortex. Aldosterone acts on the distal tubules of the kidney to increase the reabsorption of sodium (Harvey and Johns 1980:766).

The main functioning unit of the kidney is the nephron. Each kidney is made up of approximately one million nephrons. Within the nephron, filtration takes place in the glomerulus, while the tubules of the nephron are responsible for reabsorption and excretion. The main products that are normally reabsorbed are protein, glucose, amino acids and electrolytes (Gutch and Stoner 1971:26). When a significant portion of the kidney tissues are destroyed, the primary homeostatic functions of the kidney are altered. It is interesting to note that as little as one-tenth of the normal kidney function is required for life (Papper 1971:86).

Many conditions that cause acute renal failure are reversible following hemodialysis. Any acute condition that may compromise the flow to the kidney may result in acute failure. Also, certain substances that are toxic to the kidney, such as mercury, phosphorus, and some types of mushrooms, will produce acute renal failure requiring hemodialysis. Conditions that may lead to irreversible renal damage include glomerulonephritis, pyelonephritis, arteriolar nephrosclerosis (which may result from hypertension), gout, obstruction of the lower urinary tract, and hydronephrosis. These conditions may be present for years before symptoms of chronic renal failure are noted (Gutch and Stoner 1971:28–29).

Renal failure will result in uremia, which is a retention of nitrogenous products (urea, creatinine, uric acid). Carbohydrate metabolism, protein metabolism, and fat metabolism are all altered in the presence of uremia. Cardiovascular problems such as pericarditis, uremic cardiomyopathy, arrhythmias, and hypertension are often common results of uremia.

Healthy kidneys balance sodium and potassium excretion and reabsorption. This delicate balance is greatly disturbed in the presence of end stage disease. With the abnormal loss of sodium, the patient will be acidotic. An abnormal retention of sodium will result in fluid retention, which leads to edema and high blood pressure. An abnormally high serum potassium may cause muscle cramps and muscle twitching, and may lead to cardiac arrest. An elevated potassium level is quite common in patients with end stage renal disease (Gutch and Stoner 1971:30).

Anemia is the rule in end stage renal failure. When kidney tissue is damaged or destroyed, the production of erythropoietin is disturbed, leading to failure of the marrow to produce a normal quantity of red blood cells. Many hemodialysis patients require frequent transfusions. Hepatitis can be a serious complication of frequent transfusions, and dialysis personnel must be extremely cautious while handling patients' blood (Gutch and Stoner 1971:148).

Calcium metabolism is severely affected in the presence of uremia. Normal absorption of calcium from the gut is interrupted, which stimulates the parathyroids to pull calcium out of the bone in order to maintain a normal serum calcium level. This condition predisposes the patient to fractures, especially rib fractures. Long bone fractures and fractures of the vertebrae may also occur (Gutch and Stoner 1971). A high serum calcium level may lead to an increase in calcium concentration in the dermis. This condition plus the increase in uric acid seen in uremia are thought to be responsible for the pruritus so commonly experienced by these patients (Chyatte 1979:13).

Phosphate levels are increased in the presence of renal failure. As was mentioned previously, calcium absorption may be low in the presence of uremia. High phosphate levels stimulate the parathyroids to raise the calcium level by dissolving bone. Calcium phosphate crystals may form outside of bone and in soft tissues such as the heart and lungs (*SCI Manual* 1976:56).

HEMODIALYSIS

Hemodialysis involves pumping the blood through an artificial kidney, which filters out excess fluid, waste products and electrolytes. The procedure is based on the diffusion principle that a substance of high concentration will pass through a semipermeable membrane to a substance of low concentration. Also involved is osmosis—the movement of water over concentration gradients.

Various "baths" are used that are composed of electrolyte compounds, buffer and water. These dialysing fluids remove waste materials and excess fluid from the patient's blood via diffusion, osmosis, and ultrafiltration. The blood is the substance of high concentration, and the dialysing fluid represents a substance of low concentration. The physician will determine the type of dialysate to be used. At times the composition of the dialysate may be adjusted to meet the individual's needs (Chyatte 1979:16–17).

It is important to note that heparin is administered continuously during dialysis to prevent the blood from clotting while being pumped through the artificial kidney. Close monitoring of the protime is done during the procedure. The anticoagulation effect of the heparin may still be apparent for several hours after dialysis. Therefore, these patients should never receive injections during the day of dialysis (Gutch and Stoner 1971:120).

An access to the patient's bloodstream is necessary for the artificial kidney to do its work. Various types of permanent accesses have been tried. Early in hemodialysis history, metal or glass cannulas were inserted into an artery and a vein. These cannulas were removed following dialysis and the vessels tied off. The need for repetitive dialysis led to the development of a permanent access made of Teflon and silicone. This shunt was designed by Scribner and Quinton in 1960. The tubing is surgically inserted into an artery and a vein which are joined together. Ideally, the turbulent blood flow through the shunt will limit the chances of clotting. Clotting, however, is one of the more common problems associated with external shunts. There is also the ever-present danger of hemorrhaging should the shunt come apart. The patient must always carry clamps should this occur. Infection and erosion of the skin around the shunt are also dangerous complications associated with this type of access.

In 1966 the arterio-venous (A-V) fistula was developed. This technique involves surgically joining an artery to a vein without the use of foreign materials. These fistulas increase in size over a relatively short period of time with exercise and allow the use of large-bore needles or dialysis. The skin over the fistula thickens and becomes less painful to the patient when the needles are inserted. These fistulas are usually created in the patient's arm. This type of access allows complete freedom of the arm and virtually eliminates the problems of infection and clotting. The needles must be carefully inserted to prevent hematomas, as these may render the vessel difficult or even impossible to use for several days (Gutch and Stoner 1971:102–16).

WEIGHT AND FLUID CONTROL

Because excess fluid retention is often a complication of end stage renal disease, many patients must carefully monitor and restrict their fluid intake. Weighing the patient before each dialysis is necessary to determine fluid restrictions. Hourly weights are recorded during dialysis to determine the amount of ultrafiltration accomplished during the procedure (Gutch and Stoner 1971:122). Brookline Scales are used at the SCI Hemodialysis Unit at the LBVAMC. These are bed scales, which when properly used are invaluable for this purpose. The "dry" weight is obtained after dialysis. This is the person's ideal weight after waste products and excess fluid are removed. The patient is advised to gain no more than one to one and one-half pounds per day between dialyses (*SCI Manual* 1976:55).

DIET CONTROL

Due to the severe electrolyte imbalances and the buildup of waste products in the patient with end stage renal disease, a special diet is prescribed for the patient. Since protein catabolism contributes to nitrogen accumulation, the diet must be very low in protein. Prevention of tissue breakdown in the face of low protein intake must be prevented. This objective is served by a high caloric intake in the form of carbohydrates and fats. Each patient's diet is individually prescribed as to his blood chemistry and other medical problems. For example, many hemodialysis patients are hypertensive. The diets for these patients must restrict sodium as well as protein.

Chronic renal failure often results in a high serum potassium level. An imbalance of potassium may result in heart failure. The diet for this patient is usually low in potassium. This is difficult since many carbohydrates, fruits, and vegetables are high in potassium (Gutch and Stoner 1971:135–36). Also, many salt substitutes contain high quantities of potassium. It is important to know that some diuretics, such as Aldactone, block potassium excretion. Many patients with end stage renal disease receive digatalis for their congestive heart failure. Digitalis is poorly removed by dialysis, and its toxicity may become masked by an elevated potassium level or by hypocalcemia (Gutch and Stoner 1971:155).

Although dialysis does remove many waste products and aids in balancing electrolytes, the dialysis patient who indulges in foods rich in potassium and protein may feel ill post-dialysis due to the large shift of these products. More important, the patient in a state of chronic uremia risks permanent damage to other organs. Because he does feel sick most of the time, he is unable to lead as normal a life as is possible under good control. As with any diet or restriction, patient compliance is difficult. The nurse practitioner for a SCI hemodialysis unit should be well versed in these diets. She must educate the patient about all aspects of hemodialysis, but her most difficult task may be motivating this special patient to adhere to his prescribed diet. This requires time, patience and an understanding of the patient who is not only in end stage renal disease, but is also spinal cord injured (Gutch and Stoner 1971:135–37). Very recently it has been suggested that patient compliance may be improved if the patient is allowed to eat anything he wants the night before dialysis. He must follow his prescribed diet strictly for all other meals, but this occasional indulgence may improve his disposition and compliance.

PSYCHOSOCIAL COMPONENTS

It would be ideal if the SCI patient who faces maintenance hemodialysis were one who had successfully worked through all of the stages leading to interdependence and acceptance of his SCI. The impact of being paralyzed is another story, but one that cannot be ignored when discussing the SCI patient in hemodialysis.

Findings in the literature that reviews the adjustment to an SCI reveal many common components with the adjustment necessary to maintenance hemodialysis. Dependency seems to be the common denominator. Many SCI patients must become dependent on others for their care. This is a difficult adjustment to make, and often results in either overdependence (the patient becomes demanding and fearful) or underdependence (overly confident, careless, unable to accept help) (Burke and Murray 1975:80). Likewise, overdependence and underdependence have often been observed in hemodialysis patients. The patient who is overdependent may regress and become childlike when being cared for. He is often less productive than his actual potential as seen by his family and medical staff. The underdependent patient often denies his dependence on a machine and will often become anxious, depressed, and uncooperative, especially when adhering to his prescribed diet (Chyatte 1979; Levy 1974). Most patients receive dialysis three times a week for an average of four hours a day. This is both time-consuming and costly. The SCI patient may be unable to work due to his physical limitations or to find work due to the fact that jobs are scarce for anyone in a wheelchair. Transportation may be difficult for an SCI patient who is receiving outpatient hemodialysis. Those who do have jobs will often find it difficult to maintain their employment due to the time and medical factors involved. Thus, it is essential that a multidisciplinary approach be taken toward the rehabilitation of the SCI patient receiving maintenance hemodialysis.

SUBJECTIVE FINDINGS

The SCI patient who is in end stage renal disease will most likely give a history of past urinary problems, such as frequent infections, renal stones, and episodes of hematuria, and may ever report past surgical procedures involving his kidneys, ureters or bladder. The patient may be confused, so that much of the valuable information must be obtained from past medical records. The various complaints of a patient in end stage renal disease are a result of being uremic. They can include nausea, vomiting, burning sensation in the stomach area, metallic taste, dry mouth, itching, weakness, weight loss, loss of appetite, twitching, and swelling of face or lower extremities. These symptoms may occur in any combination or order (Chyatte 1979).

OBJECTIVE FINDINGS

The patient who is uremic may be mentally unclear. He will appear chronically ill and undernourished.
  Signs and symptoms by systems:

1. Skin: Poor turgor. Color may be jaundiced due to the increase of uric acid, or pale due to anemia. Edema may be present in lower extremities or face. Excoriations from the patient scratching. Ecchymosis usually on forearms, hands and shins. Dry scales.
2. Head, eye, ear, nose, throat:Breath may smell like urine. Poor dentation. Sclera may appear jaundiced due to uremia.
3. Respiration: May be deep and rapid due to acidosis. Rales or rhonchi present due to congestive heart failure.
4. Cardiac: Tachycardia. High blood pressure. May have pulsating PMI, with enlarged cardiac border.
5. Musculo-Skeletal: Muscle atrophy. Muscle twitching from calcium and potassium abnormalities.
6. Neurological: Unable to concentrate. Deep tendon reflexes decreased. (Note: Since patient is SCI, it is important to have previous documentation of his neuro status for comparison.) Motor weakness.
7. Genito-Urinary: Urine is scanty, or there may be no output (Chyatte 1979).

DIAGNOSTIC PROCEDURES

Diagnostic studies for a patient who is thought to be in end stage renal disease prior to initial dialysis will include the following:

1. SMA6 & SMA12; creatinine, magnesium, TBIC; SGPT; HAA
2. CBC with differential
3. 24-hour urine collection for creatinine clearance; C & S of urine; routine urinalysis; specific gravity
4. Arterial blood gas if patient appears short of breath
5. EKG; chest X-ray
6. KUB; ultrasound of kidneys; renal-gram and renal-scan

Note: IVP should never be done if the creatinine clearance is less than 25 ml per minute of if the serum creatinine is greater than 2.

Once maintenance dialysis has begun, the following diagnostic studies will be performed on a routine basis (*SCI Manual* 1976):

Every dialysis.................... hemotocrit
Once a week...................... protime for patients on Coumadin
Once a month.................. SMA6, SMA12, SGPT, creatine, MG TIBC, iron, HAA, CBC with differential
Every 6 months................. chest X-ray, EKG, Metabolic Bone Survey, Nerve Conduction Time, protein electrophoresis

THERAPEUTIC MANAGEMENT

The patient who is in end stage renal disease will require a blood access that will be surgically created. With his anemia, blood transfusions may be necessary if he is symptomatic. A diet should be prescribed that is low in protein, potassium and possibly sodium. It should also be high in calories, usually in the form of carbohydrates and fats. If the patient's potassium level remains elevated after dialysis, Kayexelate may be ordered. Basogel, one tablet TID, should be prescribed if the patient's phosphate level is elevated. Thiamine, Paradoxine, multivitamins and iron supplements should be ordered to improve the patient's nutritional status. If pruritus is present, a topical hydrocortisone lotion may be applied. As with any management plan for a SCI patient, skin care and prevention of pressure sores by frequent repositioning should always be included. Also, the patient's dental status should be evaluated and, if necessary, be corrected.

PATIENT EDUCATION

The patient receiving maintenance hemodialysis should have a clear understanding of the normal functions of the kidney, as well as a clear understanding of the disease. The process of hemodialysis should be explained to both patient and family. The educated and well-informed patient is more likely to comply with instructions given by the medical staff. It may also help to decrease anxiety and limit fears. Patients should be involved when planning their care. The nurse practitioner and the dietician must reinforce patients' diet instructions. They should be made aware of the possible consequences if they do not comply with their diet. They should be instructed not to miss meals. Patients are instructed never to take any medication, including vitamins and over-the-counter preparations, unless prescribed by their physician. Patients are also made aware of the increased risk of bleeding following dialysis due to the heparin used during the procedure. They should be well versed in skin care and the prevention of fractures. Patients should be instructed to report any redness, edema or irritation noted around the access site. They should also know to notify their physician before having dental work performed. They may need prophylactic antibiotics prior to any dental procedures.

5

Pain

JUNE CRABTREE and BONNIE JOHNSON

Pain, according to Taber, is the sensation felt when a person experiences discomfort, distress, or suffering. To inflict pain, according to Webster, is to make suffer or cause distress. The literature states that pain cannot be measured because a method of measurement has not been found. It is generally recognized that the feeling of pain is subjective, and the patient's description of the pain experienced should be accepted as stated.

INCIDENCE

Spinal cord–injured patients complain that they have pain below their level of injury. Some of the patients describe what they feel as "discomfort," and others describe what they feel as "pain." Most descriptions of pain state that it began after the submission of spinal shock, approximately six months following the injury (Guttman 1976). One author states that abnormal sensations have been reported by patients four years after the injury (Nepomuceno 1979). Spasticity is involved in many patients who complain of pain. Kaplan et al., in a follow-up study of pain and spasticity, found it difficult to separate the two entities. They stated that there was a great disparity in the published literature on the incidence of pain in spinal cord injuries and that the statistics vary from 7 to 50 percent. Basic terminology is confusing and differs with each author; no adequate classification is available. Pain may be minor or moderate, but does have an increased tendency to occur as time goes on (Kaplan et al. 1962).

According to Burke, who did a very extensive literature review on the incidence of pain, in one study of 47 SCI patients, 90 percent of the patients complained of diffuse, burning pains at some time following the injury. Twenty-seven percent (126 patients) of the severe cases required the consideration of active steps to be taken for relief. Other studies cited gave statistics on the incidence of pain that varied from 35 to 94 percent. Patients with cauda equina lesions seem to have the highest incidence of disabling pain. It is obvious from a literature review that pain following SCI is a varied and unpredictable experience that for some patients can be very severe (Burke 1973).

PATHOPHYSIOLOGY

Destruction of the gray matter occurs as a result of compression or cutting of the spinal cord with the resultant bleeding into the vascular parts. The level of injury is the point where alteration is prevalent and usually includes one or two segments above and below it. Roddie, William, and Wallace (1975) write, "The condition is best designated as traumatic necrosis of the spinal cord. As the lesion heals, cavitation or a gliotic focus results." The end product is irreversible damage with disordered function. Clinical manifestations are determined by type of injury to the cord and the amount of damage that has resulted. Destruction of gray matter results in damage to sensory pathways in the spinal cord and the consequent loss of sensation. This loss of sensation follows a segmental distribution according to where the injury occurred. The sensation of pain is created by neurons within the brain when an impulse is carried to it by an afferent fiber from a pain receptor, and projected to the body. The sensation of pain is blocked at the level of injury, and the message becomes distorted (Burke 1973).

Phantom sensations occur in patients with complete transection of the spinal cord or cauda equina and are reported to be in many areas below the lesion. They have been described in the legs, or to a part of the legs and feet. The phenomenon was first observed and reported in World War I, and has been extensively written about since. One of the most comprehensive and recent reports on phantom pain in paraplegics was written by Weinstein (1962). He reported three theories but gave credence to a central one. He wrote:

> Central theories attribute the presence of a phantom to cortical representation of the amputated or deafferented body parts, which possibly, through spontaneous activity or projection or of neighboring cortical regions excite the projection areas originally representative of the missing part.

Weinstein felt that the evidence for the central theory was very good. He stated that Penfield's work on phantom pain shows that the cortical representation has a direct relationship with the phantom pain, depending on the vividness and the duration of the pain. Penfield, according to Weinstein, stimulated the cortex of an amputee during a craniotomy and evoked a phantom pain of the missing part. When he surgically removed that area of the cortex the phantom pain disappeared. He also related the studies of Katz and Haber, which show a greater sensitivity of the amputated stump in comparison to the homologous contralateral regions. Weinstein felt that this greater sensitivity could result from factors that produce a denervation super-sensitivity described by a number of persons writing in the field.

The Weinstein study included a population of patients with transection of the spinal cord, cervical lesions, thoracic lesions, and lumbar lesions. The cause of injury was bullet wound, shell fragment, fracture or compression, and disease. All the patients studied had complete loss of sensation. He found that all of the patients had phantom pain of some part or another during some period after their injury. The toes and the fingers had the highest episodes of pain. The distal-sacral area had the highest episodes of phantom pain, with the frequency decreasing in the lumbar and thoracic areas. Phantom pain was also frequently found in the rectum and the buttocks. These areas are within the sacral dermatome, as are the toes.

The greatest disparity was found when he compared the chest area in the quadriplegic; half of them felt the pain constantly, and the others felt no pain at all. He concluded that in the paraplegic, the continuous phantom is apparently unrelated to the time after injury. Thirty-one percent of the patients perceived their phantoms daily, 16 percent weekly. The phantom pain appeared immediately in 53 percent; within three months in 17 percent; and after three months in 30 percent of the cases. From the great toe to the posterior thigh, tingling was the most frequent sensation, with the second reported sensation being burning. In the trunk area, burning was perceived most frequently up to the abdomen and was then perceived as pain up to the chest; tingling was found most often in the upper arm. Generally, burning was the most frequent sensation (64 percent). The second-most frequent sensation was tingling (49 percent).

The greatest frequency of the phantom pain was found in the cervical area. Thoracic was the next most frequent area, and lumbar had the least number of phantoms. Weinstein also found that age was a factor. Higher incidence of phantom pain was reported by the older patient and by the patient who had had the injury for a longer period of time. This is contrary to the amputees who report their phantom pain fades with ime.

Other sensory problems exist below the transverse lesion. When the patient has just been injured and in the early phase of complete transverse lesion, there are two sensory differences. Superficial and deep sensory messages are carried out by the posterior columns. Anterior and lateral spinothalmic or ventro- and spinocerebellar tracts are suspended at the level of transportation. The sensory loss involves touch, superficial and deep pressure, pain, itching, temperature, position and movement, vibration, two-point discrimination, and graphaesthia. After a short period of time, the borderline between the sensitive and insensitive areas of the body, which were very sharp at first, begin their compensatory overlapping. Sensory function with the distinct severance feelings becomes dissociated and distorted.

Pain and paresthesia are especially conspicuous in shoulders and arms in patients suffering complete lesions of the cervical cord (Guttman 1976). Guttman feels that the pain above the level of the lesion is the result of faulty positioning of the upper limbs in the early stages following the injury. Patients with complete transverse lesions, particularly mid-thoracic and thoraco-lumbar cord, develop a hyperpathic zone at the border and above the lesion, which may involve one or more dermatomes. It may develop into a very influential clinical symptom with complaints of band-like tightness and burning pain characteristics. A slight touch or pressure on the bedding may produce tremendous discomfort. Pain and paresthesia occur frequently in cauda equina lesions, especially partial ones. The root irritation is caused by either peri-radicular adhesions, as a result of post-traumatic arachnoiditis, or by post-traumatic changes in the damaged roots themselves (Guttman 1976).

PSYCHOSOCIAL COMPONENTS

Psychosocial makeup of individuals both before and after an injury, according to the literature, does affect the susceptibility to pain. Yet, the extent to which psychological factors play a role in the pain experience of any specific patient is a facet of assessment that is considered to be barely beyond the speculative stage (Calsyn, Louks, and Freeman 1979). Spinal cord–injured patients who were drug abusers before injury are more likely to have more pain after injury (Burke 1973).

Self-concept and body image play an extremely important role in spinal cord injuries. Physical deformity threatens body image, and disability threatens to alter dramatically the client's lifestyle. Individuals cherish and guard their wholeness; it determines their sense of security and self-esteem. The spinal cord–injured patient has his entire personality thrown off balance. He is forced to change his body concept. This transition does not occur at the time of injury, but is a lengthy process that varies with each individual. The patient may blame his failures on pain, since pain may be a more acceptable entity than loss of function (Roberts 1976). Adaptation to paralysis involves body function and becomes a tremendous threat. It inevitably involves the patient's coping mechanisms. Very often the way life was handled before the injury will provide the best prediction of behavior post-injury. Motivations to recover and return to life in the community will be strongly influenced by the presence or absence of a significant other, as well as by the family response. It is clear that a number of disciplines are needed in order to begin to cope with pain in the spinal cord–injured patient. Many spinal cord injuries require the assistance of a social worker because the patient experiences drastic economic loss from his permanent disabilities. Psychological help may also be beneficial to the nursing staff, who tend to dehumanize the patient or become discouraged when long-term care is required. Poor adjustment to the disability may be the result of continuing depressing, anger, frustration, and low self-esteem.

SUBJECTIVE AND OBJECTIVE DATA

The nonspecific subjective complaints of pain in spinal cord injury are difficult to deal with. The typical objective symptoms associated with pain are nonexistent in spinal cord injuries below their lesion. Phantom types of pain are described below the level of the lesion. The patient may complain of "heaviness," "dull aches," "fullness to the bursting point," "stabbing," "burning or busting," "tight bands," or "hot pins."

MANAGEMENT PLAN

DIAGNOSTIC

Pain varies in etiology and nature depending upon the extent or type of spinal cord injuries. Lack of sensation creates bizarre patterns. Usually there are no obvious factors for the pain; it is diffuse and not localized. It could be organic or phantom pain. A patient who has not previously complained of pain should be examined to rule out other causes of pain.

Pain clinics have been initiated in most areas with a sizable SCI population. They use a multi-treatment approach. The commonly used modalities include:

1. behavior modification
2. lifestyle change
3. use of transcutaneous electrical nerve stimulator (TENS)
4. hypnosis
5. self-hypnosis
6. biofeedback
7. relaxation techniques
8. rhizotomy.

The resources of the patient are identified and used constructively in his treatment. The patient and his or her marital partner or significant other are frequently treated together. They are usually seen weekly and progress to longer periods of time for as long as it is necessary to control the pain. The methods of treatment vary, and two or three may be used at one time.

Transcutaneous electrical nerve stimulators (TENS) are a first-line modality for most patients. If they are not effective, hypnosis will frequently be added. Hypnosis involves concentration plus imagination and suggestion. At first the patient is put in a trance, then as he relaxes and concentrates he becomes more deeply hypnotized. Imagination of water or rain falling in the woods is suggested to block the perception of the burning pain. Emotive imagery has been found to be most effective in increasing pain tolerance (Weisenberg 1979). Emotive imagery relies upon producing feelings such as self-assertion and pride. Whichever strategy is used, it must fit the person involved.

The most frequently ascribed theory for the use of the TENS is the Gate-Control Theory. This theory states that counterirritation serves to activate large-fiber activity, which through peripheral and central biasing mechanisms closes down the gate and thus blocks pain stimulation (Weisenberg 1979). Inhibition takes place when there are multiple sensory stimuli. When the TENS is placed on the skin, it competes with the other pain. It is a mental distraction. The quality of sensation is thus changed by exciting neurons in the skin. Guidelines for the use of the transcutaneous electrical nerve stimulator may be helpful for the reader unfamiliar with its use. Medical staff should:

1. Determine the location of the patient's pain.
2. Describe the features of TENS to the patient:
   a. The TENS procedure involves the mechanical placement of electrodes on the cutaneous surface of the skin, slightly above the painful region.
   b. One negative electrode and one positive electrode are placed on opposite sides of the spinal column. A battery stimulator is used. The batteries permit the passage of square waves between the two electrodes. The frequency and amplitude can be varied. Electrode placement is a trial-and-error procedure until a location is found that gives relief to the pain (Heilborn 1977/78). Inhibition takes place when there are multiple sensory stimuli.
3. Determine the best placement of electrodes:
   a. Most often placed on either side of the spinal cord, just above the level of the injury, to close the gate and block out the painful stimuli. If there is localized pain in an area where sensation exists, placement should be on either side of the painful area. Sometimes acupuncture points are used as reference for placement.
4. Activate the TENS for one hour four times per day, or when pain is especially severe.
5. Instruct the patient to keep records to determine the effectiveness of the treatment.

6. Analyze the records for use as a basis for recommendations for modification or change in therapy.

When patients are selected for treatment by the pain clinic, they are usually required to repeat the rehabilitation therapy program. This program involves the patient in a succession of obligatory activities: occupational, diversive, and functional. This repetition is necessary to help the patient deemphasize his attitude toward the pain that he must live with (Heilborn 1977/78).

Weisenberg states that it is becoming increasingly clear that pain reactions can be affected by many psychological variables, often to a much greater degree than by pharmacological means. The status of the patient, psychologically, is a determining factor regarding the effectiveness of the drug. Placebos are being used along with behavior procedures to teach patients to live with pain. Relaxation methods, hypnosis, biofeedback, emotive imagery, and several other methods are currently being utilized.

PATIENT EDUCATION

It is generally considered best to teach the patient to cope with pain after educating him in the various methods of coping. In this manner, the patient will feel in charge. One of the problems of being in a hospital is that the patient becomes depersonalized. It makes sense to put patients in charge of their pain control. One should be aware that the manner in which pain is expressed could very well be associated with ethnicity, extroversion, and introversion. Each of the foregoing types reacts to pain differently. Extroverts are thought to condition less well and therefore to develop less anxiety to the stimulation (Weisenberg 1979). Extroversion has been associated with more complaints of pain. It is believed that introverts have a higher arousal level and therefore have a lower pain threshold. Underlying attitudes and anxiety reactions appear to have a major effect on differences in pain tolerance. Some attitudes about pain are reflected in denial or avoidance of dealing with pain by persons who feel that the best way to handle pain is to ignore it. Others feel that it is a sign of weakness to give in to pain. Still others want the doctor to get rid of the pain even before they find out what the trouble is. Those who achieve success in dealing with the pain seem more highly motivated or determined to fight back (Nepomuceno 1979).

More education is needed for people who arrive at the scene of an accident first. Conservative management of the spine produces minimal scarring from the injury. Since it has been found that decompressive laminectomy for edema is really of no avail, the trend toward conservative management may decrease the pain experienced by future SCI patients.

6

Spasticity

MARY GARDENHIRE

The occurrence of spasticity is "one of man's major motor afflictions" (Bishop 1977). This is especially true if associated with spinal cord injury. Yet, there is no unanimous agreement on the exact meaning of this condition. Spasticity, as seen in spinal cord injury, is an indication that a muscle stretch reflex has become isolated from its supraspinal inhibitory-modulation system (Stryker 1972). This results in an imbalance of facilitory and inhibitory influences upon the gamma efferent neurons. The facilitory impulses entering the spinal cord from the skin, ligaments, and muscles take over. Therefore, what is seen is a heightened reflex activity, a state of hypertonicity or increase over the normal tone of muscles (Coleman 1976).

INCIDENCE AND EPIDEMIOLOGY

Epidemiological studies have shown that almost all cervical lesions have spasticity. Thoracic lesions are accompanied by spasticity 75 percent of the time, while 58 percent of the lumbar lesions and 25 percent of conus-cauda equina lesions have spasticity. Spasticity may be more severe in partial lesions, as compared with complete lesions. In incomplete lesions, voluntary motor functions are also overridden by spasticity, resulting in useless voluntary functions (Burke and Murray 1975).

Following spinal shock in an upper motor neuron lesion, signs of spasticity may appear as early as two to three months. However, the average time for the appearance of spasticity in cervical lesions is six weeks. Physical signs of spasticity in thoracic lesions may occur in ten weeks. Reflex excitability is at its maximum in two years following the injury, gradually dwindling in severity thereafter (Burke and Murray 1975).

There is no record of deaths as a result of spasticity. However, persistent underlying complications can lead to an increase in morbidity and mortality if not treated promptly and properly (Hardy and Elson 1976). To understand fully the mechanism of spasticity one must have a basic knowledge of how the muscular and nervous systems are involved physiologically.

REVIEW OF THE PHYSIOLOGY OF THE STRETCH REFLEX

The stretch reflex is important in maintaining muscular tone and producing a background of postural tone against which voluntary movement occurs.

AFFERENT ARC

When a muscle is stimulated, impulses travel to specialized receptors called muscle spindles. A muscle spindle is a small, fusiform, intramuscular structure found parallel to skeletal muscle fibers of the extrafusal fibers. They are independent of blood supply and enervation (Downey and Darling 1971). Muscle spindles are responsible for supplying the central nervous system with information about the length and velocity in changing muscle.

The transmissions from primary endings excite their own motor neuron pool and inhibit antagonistic motor neuron pools. The response to secondary endings are excitatory to flexor motor neurons and inhibitory to extensor motor neurons (Downey and Darling 1971). Other receptors of importance are the golgi tendon organs located in the tendon. These receptors transmit signals through rapidly conducting A alpha fibers. They lie in series with the extrafusal muscle fibers. Golgi tendon organs detect tension during contraction and transmit information to the motor control system of the spinal cord and cerebellum. Overall, they are associated with muscle movements, equilibrium and posture (Guyton 1971).

Internuncial cells are present in the base of the dorsal horn and anterior horn. Sensory signals are transmitted first to the internuncial cells. They are responsible for many of the integrative functions of the cord.

EFFERENT ARC

Fibers found in the efferent arc are of the gamma motor axons. They are smaller and conduct more slowly than do axons to the extrafusal muscle fibers, which are of the alpha subgroup. On the basis of nerve section size, type of motor terminal ending, threshold stimulation, and conduction velocity variations, fibers further divide into groups called gamma fibers. Gamma fibers are larger in diameter than others.

The gamma loop consists of connections to and from the spinal cord, including the muscle spindle and gamma efferent or motor fiber. The muscle spindle can be thought of as the sensory part of a reflex system that denotes differences in length between itself and the main muscle mass, acting to decrease the difference. The supraspinal control of the gamma system can be facilitory or inhibitory (Grant 1964).

The threshold excitability of the gamma motor neuron is usually lower than that of the alpha motor neuron. Consequently, under normal conditions, the gamma neurons are activated first. This is followed by discharge of the afferent sensory neurons, and finally by activation of the alpha motor neurons (Downey and Darling 1971). Descending neural impulses traveling down the spinal cord via heterogeneous tracts are concerned with

1. mediation of somatic motor activity
2. controlling muscle tone
3. suprasegmental control of reflex activity
4. enervation of viscera and autonomic structure
5. modification of sensory input (Downey and Darling 1971).

The systems and tracts are responsible for the following actions: The corticospinal tract is concerned with voluntary somatic motor function. Impulses from this system are responsible for discrete movement and form the basis for acquired motor skill. Lesions of this tract produce paralysis, alterations of muscle tone, and modifications of reflexes. The rubrospinal tract is concerned with tone in the flexor muscle group. Facilitation of flexor muscle tone occurs contralaterally to impulses descending from the motor cortex. The vestibulospinal tract exerts inhibitory influences on the cervical motor neurons. Fibers from this tract are responsible for autonomic responses (Downey and Darling 1971).

The extrapyramidal motor system involves the upper motor neurons, which travel to lower motor neurons via paths other than the pyramidal tract. The pyramidal system is involved in the initiation of voluntary movements, whereas the extrapyramidal system is responsible for providing a suitable background of muscle tone and posture for those movements. This tract is also concerned with execution of voluntary movement and suppression of involuntary movement. Overall, the physiological mechanism of this system is not fully understood. If it is damaged, however, certain clinical signs are seen (Roddie, William, and Wallace 1975).

Inhibition and facilitation play an important part in the firing or decrease in firing of neurons. Facilitory tracts act by decreasing the resisting potential of the lower motor neuron to its threshold of stimulation. Facilitory impulses tend to increase the tone of extensor muscles and decrease the tone of flexor muscles. Inhibitory impulses increase the lower motor neuron membrane potential above its resting level. They inhibit the lower motor neuron to extensor muscles and stimulate those of flexor muscles (Roddie, William, and Wallace 1975).

Basic physiology has been reviewed to acquaint the reader with the complexity of stretch reflexes at the segmental level. It is important to remember that muscle tone is regulated by the corticospinal tract, which accompanies the pyramidal tract in exerting a tonic inhibitory effect on the stretch reflex. This inhibition is balanced by the constant background facilitation from the reticulospinal and vestibulospinal pathways to provide the degree of muscle tone needed for voluntary movement. These descending motor pathways are influenced threefold by the brainstem, cerebellum, and basal ganglia in gaining control (Lance 1974).

THE MECHANISM OF SPASTICITY

Whenever the flow of neuronal impulses is interrupted at any point along the pathway from reception to motor response, an alteration in motor response occurs. This functional alteration may be expressed as a sensory, motor, or sensory and motor disturbance, depending on the location of the neuronal interruption.

For thousands of years it has been recognized that a combination of hypertonus and muscular paresis could be caused by damage or disease of the central nervous system. It was not until the end of the nineteenth century, however, that this disordered function and its correlation with specific lesions within the brain and spinal cord were recognized. It was pointed out by Dr. H. Jackson that a nerve lesion cannot produce anything but a loss of some function. Therefore, by taking the cerebral influence from the anterior horns, the cerebellar influence on them is no longer antagonized (Rushworth 1964). This leads to facilitory impulses entering the spinal cord from the skin, ligaments and muscle to predominate (Lance 1974). What we then see in motor signs are the following:

1. Stretch reflexes that are normally latent become obvious.
2. Tendon reflexes (i.e., the phasic reflexes) have a lowered threshold to tap.
3. The response of the tapped muscle is increased.
4. Muscles, other than those tapped, usually respond.
5. Tonic stretch reflexes (i.e., resistance to passive movement) are similarly affected.
6. Clonus may be produced (Bishop 1977).

Because several of the motor signs occur as a result of transection of the pyramidal tract, a brief description will be given of the descending pathway responsible for spasticity. If there is a lesion of the pyramidal tract (part of the descending pathway), one will see most of the clinical signs listed above. This lesion may sometimes be referred to as an upper motor neuron lesion, as previously stated (Roddie, William, and Wallace 1975).

Irritation to this tract also gives rise to an increase in the traffic of impulses, and uncontrolled muscular contractions and spasticity result. In spasticity, the reflex arc is devoid of its supraspinal modulation system and is, therefore, performing as a hyperactive reflex in isolation. Due to this shortcircuiting of the normal regulating system, there is abnormal excitability of alpha and dynamic fusimotor neurons. If there is any irritation to the dorsal reticulospinal system, flexor reflex afferent pathways are disinhibited (Lance 1974). This disinhibition causes the stretch reflexes of the lower limb to respond in the following manner: (a) velocity-dependent excitation of the tonic stretch reflex in flexors and extensors, and (b) length-dependent facilitation of flexor muscles and inhibition of extension muscles. This is known as the "clasp knife" phenomenon (Lance 1974).

Of primary concern is the patient with complete transection of the spinal cord. This patient has a release of flexor reflexes from brain stem control. Flexor spasticity can then easily occur in response to stimulation of cutaneous, bladder, or bowel afferents. Care of this particular patient should be taken to avoid paraplegia-in-flexion, which may occur when the hips and knees are severely flexed (Hardy and Elson 1976). Lance (1974) states that in the upper limbs the difference between the effect of flexor reflex afferents on flexor and extensor motorneurons is less apparent.

One must remember that the isolated segment of the cord can be stimulated by almost any source of irritation in the lower limb. Such irritation is called afferent stimulation. A reflex arc develops and spasticity constitutes its efferent component. When exaggerated or new spasticity occurs in a previously stabilized patient, the underlying cause should be investigated and corrected. Important examples of efferent stimuli as listed by Hardy and Elson (1976) are:

1. sensory stimulation from a distended bladder
2. sensory stimulation from a distended bowel
3. sensory irritation from a pressure sore
4. sensory irritation from contractures
5. sensory irritation from bed clothes, wearing apparel, or badly fitting appliances
6. emotional upset.

PSYCHOSOCIAL IMPACT OF SPASTICITY

Spasticity impacts on a person's self-esteem and interpersonal relationships. Guttman (1973) has written:

A disaster in human life of such magnitude as a sudden transection or severe injury to the spinal cord, which throws the body completely out of gear, inevitably disrupts the psychophysical entity of the organism resulting in pronounced effects on the paralyzed patient's mind.

In considering psychosocial aspects of spasticity one must ascertain the existing personality of the paralyzed patient before the injury. This provides a more complete picture of the patient's personality and enables one to predict the reaction to this sudden life change. The change in the appearance or body image is overwhelming to the patient. The constant tap of a spastic limb is most annoying. The attending staff must realize what is going on and try to reassure the patient (Hardy and Elson 1976). It should be emphasized to patients and their families that spasticity is neither a good nor a bad prognostic sign. Attempting to convince them that this movement is not related to gaining control of the paralyzed part is a difficult task, and should be approached cautiously (Howe 1977). Patients may or may not alert the nurse to their awareness of this new movement; they may be too afraid to ask questions. One can be sure, however, that the patient is aware of these movements.

The severity of spasticity varies from mild, through moderate, to severe. Its occurrence may present no problem and occasionally may be advantageous. Some patients use spasticity for transferring, walking, and putting on clothes. Involuntary movements during sexual intercourse can either be advantageous or disadvantageous. Without this spasticity, extremities are limp and useless in sustaining an erection. Hence, there will either be enjoyment, or disgust and lowered self-esteem. Staff caring for patients experiencing spasticity should make the patient aware of his capabilities by utilizing and developing his abilities. The staff should also assist the patient in the identification of his limitations and making plans to compensate for them.

OBJECTIVE ASSESSMENT DATA

The physical examination of the patient will reveal the following findings, according to Davis (1975).

1. The examiner may first notice that the patient is either spastic or not. Other than the fact of the spinal cord injury, all other information on disposition will vary according to the presenting causes of hospitalization and severity of spasticity.

2. By the second month after injury, the skeletal motor reflex arcs are sensitive to muscle stretch reflex if stimulated and if sustained clonus is seen.

3. The examiner will elicit flexor limb withdrawal to the slightest cutaneous stimulation-mass reflex.

4. By the end of the third month after injury, the examiner will see generalized spasticity and increased excitability of the reflex system.

5. There will be noticeable increased spasticity below the level of injury.

6. Hyperactivity of the deep tendon reflex can be elicited.

7. The H-reflex (electrical stimulation of the posterior tibial nerve) recovers faster in spastic patients as opposed to normal subjects. This indicates increased central excitability.

8. There can be a general enhancement of all phasic muscle reflexes leading to the reflex spread or irradiation. This phenomenon occurs when a vibratory wave propagates from a point of percussion, triggering off tendon jerks by stimulating spindles of all muscles in the path of the vibratory wave. For example, one may notice the H-reflex elicited elsewhere in the musculature, not previously recorded. This can be due to hypersensitivity or axonal sprouting.

9. The examiner may not be able to elicit a deep tendon reflex if spasticity is severe. This is due to the high tonic stretch reflex.

10. The examiner may see signs of one reflex system influencing the others. For example, the stimulus coming from an infected pressure ulcer in the skin could cause an increase in the tone of all muscles, especially the flexor group.

11. The examiner should be aware that spasticity increases as the level of mental stress increases.

12. A classical sign noted in spastic patients is the "clasp knife" phenomenon.

For proper treatment to occur, the clinician must first distinguish spasticity from other clinical disorders with similar signs:

1. *Ridigity* differs from spasticity in that there is a relatively constant resistance throughout range of motion (Grant 1964). This can be due to an extrapyramidal tract lesion.
2. *Athetosis* is a fluctuation in posture of variable speed and magnitude affecting the hands and, less often, the feet (Lane 1964).
3. *Dystonia* is a fixed posture in which passive stretch results in an increasing "springy" resilience (Lane 1964).
4. *Clonus* is seen when contraction and relaxation of muscle alternate in rapid succession.
5. A *contracture* is a thickening and shortening of connective tissue resulting in limited movement. It usually occurs as a result of improper management of spasticity.

Investigations have concluded that some of these intermingling symptoms do not respond to antispasmolytic medication. Therefore, Leavitt and Wells (1964) feel one should "identify in detail the facets of the disease state presented in a given case. Such documentation, of course, has, in the final analysis, a direct bearing on evaluation of treatment effects."

MANAGEMENT PLAN

DIAGNOSTIC PLAN

Treatment of spasticity needs to be based on the classical concept of the underlying neural mechanism. Patients presenting identical clinical signs may have various underlying neural causes of spasticity. Proper diagnosis of spasticity must be made before any treatment can be initiated (Bishop 1977). Some experimental tests have been developed to detect and analyze excitatory excess and inhibitory deficits leading to abnormal motor signs and spasticity. Preliminary results indicate the tests may have an important role in diagnosis and treatment of spasticity in the future. Bishop (1977) describes the tests as (a) quantitative measure of the tonic and phasic stretch reflexes to determine the relative contributions of the static and hynamic gamma systems to the excitatory excess giving rise to the hyperactive reflexes; (b) suppression of the tonic vibration reflex; and (c) irradiation of reflex responses.

A second requirement necessary before the clinician can initiate proper treatment is assessing a patient's state of recovery. It has been documented that after a lesion, the patient may gain some return in function. Formerly, recovery was documented as a result of reunion of temporarily impaired neural systems. Other additional phenomena attributed to gainful function are

> adaptive changes in existing neural networks, formation of new synaptic connections, reorganization of existing neural networks, and functional compensation through substitution induced by retraining. Each phenomenon promises to have a profound influence on the way patients with motor disturbances will be managed in the future

THERAPEUTIC PLAN

The aim of treatment of the spastic patient is to decrease the afferent limb of the reflex perpetrating the muscle contraction. The practitioner should remove or treat any irritant foci that might cause afferent stimuli. Bishop (1977) believes that a patient responds dramatically with temporary relief of flexor spasm when the placebo effect is initiated. This is done when there is an intervention between the patient and a sympathetic friend, doctor, or therapist. The placebo effect should be used in all treatment management. One should remember never to promise the patient normal function, but to teach use of what function remains.

Therapeutic exercises have several desired outcomes. These include improvement of range of motion, strengthening of voluntary control, reduction of unwanted muscular activity, and gaining maximum use of remaining function. It is important that the spastic limb be put through range of motion at least twice daily (Burke and Murray 1975). The therapist should massage the affected limb to maintain muscle tone. Hydrotherapy using the Hubbard tank relieves muscle spasticity, decreases pain, increases circulation, and improves muscle tone. Water exercises also give the patient a sense of well-being, a feeling of independence and free movement. Cooling of the spastic limb has proven effective in the treatment of spasticity. Local cooling increases the excitability of the alpha motor neurons while inhibiting the gamma motor neuron (Beland 1972).

When the patient is able, standing and walking should be encouraged to aid in the flexor pattern and circulation, and to decrease bladder complications. Research has shown that a spastic patient can be strapped to a bicycle to exercise his extremities. Positive results include an increase in circulation, muscular tone and joint mobility (Davis 1975). The paralyzed limb should be positioned carefully each time the patient is turned. For example, if the patient is being turned laterally, the upper limb is kept fully extended at the hip and knee. The foot is placed firmly in a neutral position against a foot board at the end of the bed (Hardy and Elson 1976). If tolerated, the patient should be placed in the prone position, as it holds the lower limbs fully extended. The patient should be repositioned every two hours. The flexor pattern predisposes one to contracture (Burke and Murray 1975). In incomplete lesion, the practitioner may find some advantages in using EMG biofeedback. This procedure has shown gainful control of spasticity and improved functional ability of the paralyzed limb (Baker and Reyenas 1977).

Drugs

The ideal drug would be one that relieves spasticity with minimal side effect. As of today, there is no drug that accomplishes this effect. The following are some of the drugs currently used to relieve or decrease spasticity.

1. *Lioresal* (Baclofen) decreases spasticity through action at the spinal level inhibiting monosynaptic reflexes. It is used for painful spasticity as well as for relief of flexor spasm, clonus, and muscular rigidity. The dosage should be titrated as follows: 5 mg three times daily for three days, 10 mg three times daily for three days, 15 mg three times daily for three days, and 20 mg three times daily for three days. Total dosage should not exceed 80 mg daily.
2. *Diazepam* (Valium) has a relevant effect on spasticity if given in small dosages. If used for a prolonged period, it can lead to addiction. Alcohol is contraindicated when Valium is used. The main side effect is drowsiness and fatigue.

3. *Dantrolene sodium* (Dantrium) is an anti-spasmodic drug that works on the muscle itself. The exact mechanism is unknown, but it is believed to interfere with the role of calcium in muscular contraction. Adverse reactions include drowsiness, dizziness, nausea and vomiting. This drug has been used to decrease spasticity accompanied by pain (Dykes 1975). It is sometimes combined with Diazepam, since the combination of the two drugs appears more effective than either alone (Glass 1974).

4. Other drugs that may be used include Curare, Myanesen, Chlormezzanine, Equanil, Flexine, and Physestimine (Coleman 1976). All of these drugs in some way decrease motor neuron function by acting centrally on facilitory areas.

Surgical Procedures

Numerous surgical procedures have been used to relieve spasticity. This mode of treatment needs to be carefully evaluated against the possible damage to the patient's functioning ability. Selection of procedure depends on the degree and type of spasticity. Studies have reported the return of voluntary control as late as two years. It is therefore recommended that consideration of any surgical procedure be postponed until after this time (Howe 1977). The surgical procedures are as follows:

1. Division of tendon and muscles (*tenotomy* or *myotomy*). This procedure is elected for patients who have plantar flexor contractures (Guttman 1973). The strong flexors of the hip and knee can be divided. At the ankle, the tendo-achilles can be lengthened to collect spastic flexion of the feet. The idea is to decrease the amount of spasticity without abolishing it (Burke and Murray 1975).

2. Division of nerves (*neurotomy*) involves sectioning of the obturator nerves for relief of adduction spasm. This scissoring type of spasticity interferes with walking and administration of nursing care.

3. *Tendon transplantation* for the correction of severe spastic pes-equinovarus (a deformity of the foot where the heel is elevated and turned inward and the foot is turned down) by transferring part of the whole of the tibialis anterior tendon onto the extensor digitorium.

4. *Rhizotomy* is a very complicated procedure, mainly because root identification is difficult. Patients should be given a chance to weigh the pros and cons of having this operation. Posterior rhizotomy is sectioning of the posterior roots of the spinal nerves. Guttman (1973) reports return of spasticity in several subjects. This is because the impulses from the remaining roots eventually compensate for the lost afferent impulses of the divided roots. An anterior rhizotomy is indicated for intractable spasticity. However, this procedure turns the spastic limb into a lower motor neuron

lesion. It destroys the reflex arc, predisposing the patient to loss of bowel, bladder, and sex functioning, and precludes the miracle of walking (Beland 1972).

5. A *myelotomy* is a difficult procedure to perform. It is indicated for lower limb spasticity. It breaks the reflex arc by selectively dividing the connections between the anterior and posterior horns.

6. *Chordotomy* or *chordectomy* involves resection of several segments. This procedure is hardly ever performed, mainly because it abolishes reflex activity of bowel, bladder and sex functions.

7. A *motor point block* uses diluted phenol solution injected into motor end points. Here, the gamma motor fibers are blocked; therefore, the muscle spindles are blocked. This causes the muscle spindles to be less responsive to stretch. The effect is temporary, rarely lasting longer than two weeks (Guttman 1973).

8. A *subarachnoid block* converts an upper motor neuron to a lower motor neuron by demyelination of the spinal roots. It is indicated for generalized excessive spasticity of the legs. This block destroys sacral sparing, for the alcohol has a permanent effect as opposed to phenol (Burke and Murray 1975).

9. The insertion of a *peroneal nerve stimulator* increases muscular bulk and decreases spasticity (Davis 1975).

10. *Distilled water* may be injected percutaneously into the cord. It creates a cyst between the cord and the anterior horn that interferes with the reflex arc, causing a decrease in spasticity (Davis 1975).

11. One of the latest means of treating spasticity surgically is by the *percutaneous radiofrequency thermal selective sensory rhizotomy*. In this procedure, thermal lesions are made at the dorsal root ganglion. Here, the small, sensory unmyelinated fibers will be destroyed while the heavily myelinated motor fibers remain intact. The destruction of the unmyelinated fibers decreases facilitory impulses, therefore greatly decreasing spasticity (Coleman 1976).

PATIENT EDUCATION

Areas of patient education have been discussed throughout this chapter. Here are some of the important points:

1. The patient, as well as the patient's family, should have an understanding of the overall mechanism of spasticity.

2. The patient should be taught to use spasticity to his advantage. Some examples include (a) allowing spasticity to aid in transferring, standing and ambulating; (b) pinching of the calves of the legs causing a flexion reflex, thereby aiding in dressing of the lower extremities; (c) using move-

ments caused by spasticity to enhance the sexual relationships; (d) rubbing the abdominal skin or thighs to produce emptying of the bladder.

3.   The patient should be taught how to perform range of motion exercises and the importance of attending rehabilitative therapy.

4.   The patient should be informed of all the various stimuli that can cause spasticity.

5.   Safety measures should be reviewed, especially strapping the spastic patient in a wheel chair to avoid sliding out during episodes of spasticity.

7

Skin Breakdown

SUSAN GROGAN, KATHLEEN MORTON, and
MARGARET MURPHY

Healthy skin is dependent on the circulatory system, which moves blood and carries oxygen and nutrients to the cells and waste products away. Cells are bathed in a fluid that is separated from the external environment by semipermeable membranes. To meet the needs of the cells, material must be transported to and from these membranes. This is accomplished by a system of vessels. Arteries leave the heart and approach the tissues, branching into progressively smaller vessels. Eventually they form the microscopic structures called capillaries, in which the transportation of nutrients through the semipermeable membranes takes place. Blood moves through the tubing of the circulatory system and reaches the capillaries carying oxygen and nutrients, which pass out of the capillary and into the cell. Waste products from the cell pass into the capillaries and are returned to the heart by the venous part of the circulatory system (Martin et al. 1981).

The most crucial function of the cutaneous blood flow is nourishment of the skin, but this process can be disrupted by external pr ssure that constricts blood flow. Ischemia, or interference in the satisfactory blood supply to the tissue, results if pressure is exerted that is greater than the relatively low hydrostatic pressure of the capillaries. The blood flow and exchange of oxygen and nutrients is impeded when the blood pressure cannot overcome other pressure exerted against it.

INCIDENCE, ETIOLOGY, AND PATHOPHYSIOLOGY

Pressure sores are defined as skin and subcutaneous tissue necrosis over bony prominences from unrelieved pressure sufficient to p event adequate circulation. Synonyms are decubitus ulcers and bedsores. It is estimated that well over half the spinal cord–injured persons develop at least one pressure sore in their lifetimes. Studies conducted at Bellevue Hospital in

New York demonstrated that 42 percent of their spinal injury patients required hospitalization for treatment of pressure sores. The highest incidence is seen in the paraplegic rather than the quadriplegic population, and this diagnosis is the leading cause of prolonged hospital stay in the patient with spinal cord injury. In 1966, it was estimated that each decubitus ulcer increased the cost of the health care program by an average of $5000.00, and health care costs have increased four- or fivefold since that time (Berecek 1975).

The underlying cause of all pressure sores is unrelieved pressure for a period of time. There is a definite pressure:time relationship in the evolution of pressure sores. Skin can tolerate a minute pressure indefinitely, whereas greater pressure for a short period of time causes disruption. With the usual pressure from body weight, microscopic tissue changes secondary to local ischemia can be seen in less than 30 minutes if the pressure is sustained. Although arterial blood pressure may be 120 mmHg, this is reduced to 13–22 mmHg in the capillary bed. Maintenance of pressure greater than 35–34 mmHg will prevent adequate tissue oxygenation. Local anoxia develops and there is an increase in tissue metabolites from disruption of the return venous flow. Edema develops, which further embarrasses tissue nourishment, and the end result is death of tissues. Relief of pressure allows perfusion of tissues, removal of toxic materials, and restoration of nutrition.

In the normally enervated individual, pain secondary to nerve ending stimulation by anoxia and local chemical irritation encourages early position change with minimal cell damage. The paralyzed individual is unable to recognize these signs and fails to move frequently, resulting in tissue injury. Studies have demonstrated that tissue changes are reversible if pressure, which interferes with tissue perfusion, does not persist for longer than two hours.

Clinically there are four stages in the evolution of a pressure sore, as described by Edberg (1973). The earliest sign is a condition known as *reactive hyperemia.* When pressure has been sustained for 30 minutes or less and then relieved by turning or change in position, the patient's skin will appear reddened and warm a the point of pressure. This redness is created as blood rushes back into the newly reopened blood vessels, and usually disappears in less than one hour. This increased blood flow is sufficient to nurture the oxygen-deprived tissues and reverse any damage sustained to this point. If pressure is not relieved within two to six hours, *tissue destruction* occurs secondary to ischemia. With tissue ischemia, the pressure points again appear reddened with relief of pressure, but this redness persists for up to 36 hours.

Necrosis develops if pressure persists for more than six hours. At this stage of sore development, there may be a lump or a bluish appearance to the skin. *Ulceration,* the final stage of sore development, occurs within two weeks of the tissue necrosis. The ulcerative process begins at the epidermis because it is the thinnest layer of skin, and progresses inward to the subcutaneous and underlying tissues. This inward spread of ulceration occurs as the inflammatory process begins and edema from blood and fluid infiltration into soft tissue increases. This edema further compromises tissues by creating pressure on more blood vessels, causing them to collapse and become occluded, and leading to even further ulceration.

The location of pressure sores depends on where the patient spends the most time. When the patient is primarily in bed, sacral and lateral trochanteric lesions are common. If greater time is spent in the wheelchair, then ischial pressure sores are more common. The heels, malleoli, iliac crest, and knees are less common sites. Tissue covering the sacrum is of lesser density than other areas; therefore pressure sores in this region can easily expose the sacral bones. Skin of the trochanter region overlies a thin muscle, which is enclosed in two layers of fascia. When the muscle layer is penetrated, healing is very difficult. During hip movements of flexion or extension, the ulcer rides back and forth over the prominence of the greater trochanter, and this action does not promote healing. Overlying the ischii is specialized weight-bearing soft tissue consisting of coarse fibrous septa which enclose large fat cells. This provides a cushion between bony protruberance of the ischii and the skin. When sores in this area heal by granulation or secondary intention, a tough adherent scar forms and reduces or eliminates the cushion effect of the tissues. This scar may need to be replaced with healthier tissue and/or the ischial prominence planed down to a flatter surface so that weight on the skin is more evenly distributed.

There are two major types of skin breakdown—the superficial sores that begin at the skin surface with maceration of devitalized skin, and the deep sores that do not originate at the skin. Indeed, they are considered to be the result of a process that begins in deep tissues and spreads to the surface. Degeneration can be taking place at tissue levels from bone to skin (Berecek 1975). Clinical awareness may occur only when the skin becomes inflamed or induration develops to an extent that can be felt at the surface.

A number of other factors also contribute to skin breakdown, although prolonged pressure is the most significant. Shearing forces can play an essential part in determining the size of a developing decubitus ulcer. Shearing forces stretch and slide layers of tissue and contribute to areas of undermining surrounding decubiti. An example of shearing can be seen in a patient who develops a sacral decubitus from prolonged back-lying in bed. Both the amount and duration of the pressure of the sacrum on the bed have overcome the capillary pressure and interfered with cell nutrition enough to cause necrosis. But the direction of the pressure that has been applied, for example, when the head of the bed is elevated and body weight is shifted in a dragging, stretching manner, damages a wider tract of tissue. Patients practicing transfer skills or patients with significant spasticity may also encounter tissue damage from shearing and friction (Miller and Sachs 1974). Friction refers to surface, epidermal injury, whereas shearing involves deeper injury because of stress on fascia and vessels.

Any break in the integrity of the skin surface, either from friction, mechanical injury, burn, or pressure, predisposes the area to infection, edema, and moisture collection. Episodes of fever or other acute conditions increase the metabolic rate of the body and increase the demand for oxygen. The supply of oxygen in the patient with skin at risk is already compromised, and acute conditions increase the likelihood for breakdown and indicate that previously established safe skin times will not now be effective. This is often demonstrated when the skin of a febrile patient will not withstand the length of time in one position that had previously been determined to be safe.

Moisture, from perspiration or incontinence, reduces the resistance of the skin to other physical factors and contributes to the risk of skin breakdown. This factor is closely related to hygiene. The same patient population that is at risk for skin breakdown often has impaired bowel and bladder function. They are often dependent to some degree in maintaining hygiene and require particular attention to the perineal area. Inadequate hygiene contributes to increased bacterial population of the skin. Infecting bacteria tend to localize in ischemic tissue and increase the rapidity with which an ulcer develops.

Poor general nutrition is a factor in tissue maintenance. A negative nitrogen balance almost always accompanies bodily injury, and its severity increases with the severity of the insult. Protein loss from drainage from Grade III or Grade IV sores can be a great as 50 grams per day. Whenever edema is present, the distance from the capillary to the cell is increased. This is another source of interference in the nourishment of the skin and increases the likelihood of skin breakdown (Martin et al. 1981). The SCI patient has additional risk factors not found in the general population at risk for skin breakdown. These include:

1. *Absent Sensation.* Because most SCI patients lack normal enervation, especially in the buttock and lower extremities, they fail to sense the tingling, numbness, or pain warning them of local tissue ischemia and the need to change position.

2. *Excessive Spasticity.* While mild spasticity is beneficial in SCI in presenting muscle atrophy, excessive spasticity creates abrasions and shear-stress damage to the skin as it is rubbed against bedding, clothing, and wheelchair parts.

3. *Areflexia.* Areflexia leads to severe muscle wasting, thereby decreasing the vitality of resistance of tissues supplied by the affected nerves (Pinel 1976).

4. *Maceration.* Maceration of the skin occurs in SCI secondary to incontinence of bowel and bladder and also due to a phenomenon of excessive perspiration below the level of injury (Gruis 1976).

5. *Decrease in Vasomotor Control.* This leads to diminished vascular tone and a decrease in capillary pressure. Therefore, the intensity of pressure needed to occlude the vessels of these patients is even less than that of normal individuals (Pierce 1971).

6. *Trauma.* Lack of voluntary control over lower extremities predisposes SCI patients to an increased risk of trauma to a limb when transferring or riding in the wheelchair. This trauma can lead to hematoma, edema, and resultant tissue ischemia.

7. *Scar Tissue.* Many SCI patients with past history of sores have extensive scar tissue formation, and the ability of this tissue to withstand any pressure is greatly reduced. As a result, those patients are at very high risk for future sore development.

Pressure sores are classified on a grading system of I to IV, which serves as a guide for treatment and prognosis (El torai 1977). The most superficial presentation of a Grade I pressure sore is an irregular, ill-defined area of soft tissue swelling and induration with associated heat and erythema over a bony prominence. The extreme of Grade I involvement is a moist, superficial, irregular ulceration limited to epidermis, exposing the underlying dermis and resembling an abrasion.

Grade II is wider and deeper, penetrating through the full thickness of the dermis to the junction of subcutaneous fat. Clinically, this ulcer presents as a shallow, full thickness ulcer whose edges are more distinct, with early fibrosis and pigmentation changes blending into an indistinct area of heat, erythema, and induration.

In Grade III there is progression into subcutaneous fat where extensive undermining occurs. The epidermis thickens and rolls over the edge toward the ulcer base. An intense reactive fibrosis, inflammation, and retraction of both dermis and subcutaneous fat distort any tissue distinctions. The deep fascia is relatively avascular and physically resistant, which limits penetration of the necrotic process and encourages peripheral spread and undermining. The muscle is not directly involved but is distorted by swelling and inflammation. Clinicially, Grade III is the classical decubitus ulcer, extending into subcutaneous fat with a necrotic base that is usually draining, infected, and foul-smelling. Protein, the raw material for cellular growth, is lost in the drainage from pressure sores.

Clinical presentation of Grade IV sores resembles the previous grade, except that bone can be identified at the base of the ulcer. There is more profuse drainage, undermining, and necrosis. Bone involvement usually includes osteomylitis. If osteomylitis is long standing, amyloidosis develops, which is life-threatening and for which there is no cure. Protein loss occurs at a greater rate than can be compensated for by diet.

Pressure sores have definite phases of healing: the exudative, phagocytic, and reparative. The exudative phase is a period of acute inflammatory reaction with erythema, edema and polymorphonuclear response to soft tissue destruction. When the inflammatory response is prolonged by the presence of bacteria, the physiological response becomes very complex and includes mediated immune responses that can produce tissue injury beyond that caused by the ulcer.

The phagocytic phase represents a period of microscopic debridement and the formation of granulation tissue. During this phase the conditions responsible for soft tissue necrosis have been eliminated and the body is attempting to repair the damage that has been done. The reparative phase represents the body's attempt at reepithelialization of the tissue that has been destroyed. A number of factors influence epithelial repair. Extensive scab formation and protein deficiency inhibit repairs. Usually this area of repair will be void of hair follicles and sweat glands.

PSYCHOSOCIAL COMPONENTS

The majority of all pressure sore research, prevention, and treatment deals mainly with physical rather than psychosocial aspects associated with pressure sores. If it were purely a mechanical entity, then it stands to reason that the numerous prevention modalities available would be adequate in abolishing the existence of almost all pressure sores. The frequency and number of repeated sores, however, indicate that attention to only the mechanical factors is not enough. Therefore, when dealing with pressure sores in the SCI patient, close attention must be paid to the psychosocial components associated with pressure sore development.

Unfortunately, not much documented research is available on psychosocial factors associated with pressure sores. One study (Anderson 1979) did find a significant correlation between the incidence of pressure sores and three variables:

1. the responsibility the patient has in his own skin care,
2. the patient's satisfaction with the activities of life, and
3. to a lesser degree, the patient's self-esteem.

It was found that those patients with a high degree of responsibility for their skin care and a high satisfaction with life had a very low incidence of pressure sores. Those who had assistance with care (shared responsibility) and a low satisfaction with life had a much higher incidence of sore development.

In addition to the above-named items, several other psychosocial factors that appear to be present in many SCI patients may contribute to pressure sore development.

1. *Fatalistic attitude.* This attitude may result in passive acceptance by patients that sores are an inevitable consequence of disability. Patients feel that nothing they can do will make a difference one way or another with sores.

2. *Passivity.* During the acute stage of SCI, it is required that patients be passive; they must depend on health care personnel for their total care. If, however, during the course of rehabilitation, they are not encouraged to become more independent, they may remain in the same passive state. They may feel their care and the esponsibility of sore prevention belongs to someone else. Unless they have extremely conscientious round-the-clock aids, these patients are at risk for skin breakdown.

3. *Poor self-concept.* Throughout the course of the disorder, the progress SCI patients make depends largely on how they perceive themselves, what they think they can become, and how they see opportunities and limitations in the world around them. If they view their body images as poor, their futures as bleak, their opportunities as nil, and limitations as overwhelming, they are apt to be very depressed and noncompliant with treatment. These patients are at very high risk for sore development and may exhibit suicidal tendencies.

4. It has been hypothesized that a phenomenon known as the "Spinal Cord Personality" exists in patients with SCI. The average patient, according to this hypothesis, is "a high-risk taker, tends to act rather than contemplate, has poor personality control, limited channels for emotional expression and tends to express his aggression directly" (Ruge 1969). The only way for them to exercise any power is through verbal affronts and by noncompliance with treatment modalities. These patients may get sores not because they really want them, but because they may view it as the only way to show that they are still in charge and don't have to conform to the rules of others.

5. *Inadequate support system.* Patients who have no strong family ties or significant others tend to develop sores more frequently than those patients who have good support systems. Patients who have no one to assist them with their care or to voice an interest in their well-being may feel very alone and lacking in self-worth. They may become depressed and, as a result, negligent in their care.

Once a pressure sore has developed, the psychosocial impacts on the patient are numerous. At best, pressure sore development is time-consuming and costly, but at worst, it can lead to debilitating systemic conditions and even death. In a patient whose self-concept is already poor, the possibility of further scarring, disfiguration, or even amputation from pressure sores would be devastating. Pressure sores, many times, cause patients to be removed from their jobs, families, and social settings due to hospitalization. They may be required to forfeit many common activities of daily living such as sitting in their wheelchairs and managing their own bowel care. If the sore becomes infected, they may have to suffer the loneliness and boredom of isolation. Many times the dignity and privacy of patients are forgotten as they are subjected to frequent dressing changes and surgical rounds where they are viewed and discussed by numerous health personnel. If patients must bear the cost of their own treatment, they may be faced with a heavy financial burden due to prolonged stays in the hospital. Even under the best of conditions, sores are a very frustrating and discouraging occurrence to most patients.

Four stages of adjustment for the person who has suffered a spinal injury have been documented (Rigoni 1971):

1. *Shock.*   The patient appears totally overcome by the disability. He does not seem aware of his surroundings or what is being done for him.
2. *Defensive Retreat.*   The most common psychological phenomenon at this stage is denial. The patient refuses to believe he is paralyzed and will never be able to walk again.
3. *Acknowledgment.*   The patient internalizes awareness of the true extent of his disability. This period is characterized by depression and grief.
4. *Coping Phase.*   The patient begins to adapt and make changes in order to adjust to his environment. He shows heightened interest in relearning activities that were second nature to him prior to injury.

Depression, denial and frustration are the most common behaviors exhibited during and after the adjustment period. Frustration causes emotional reactions such as hostility, anger, uncooperativeness, and acting out. Denial extends to being inattentive to essential self-care, which can result in pressure sores. Depression characterizes itself by not caring what happens to the body. Pressure sores may be an additional insult that strains the patient's coping mechanisms in any stage of adjustment. How patients deal with pressure sores is greatly influenced by their pas coping experiences. Even though a sore is a major setback, if they have developed adequate coping skills, the patients will learn to adapt and to survive. If coping skills are poor, a pressure sore can be another major catastrophe in their lives.

The impact of a patient's pressure sores on the family can vary. Some families take it in stride with little disruption. With others, it inflicts utter chaos. If the patient is hospitalized, this separation causes family roles and interactions to change. Hospitalization, or the possible loss of a job, may place the family in grave financial distress. Whereas the patient may have been the primary breadwinner before, some other family member may be forced into that position during the patient's absence. There may be a sense of guilt, anger, or resentment on the part of the family. They feel guilty that they might possibly have been able to prevent the sore; angry with the patient for developing the sore; and resentment that their lives have been disrupted because of the sore. Conversely, some families might view the separation with relief because they are free, at least temporarily, from the cumbersome duties of caring for the patient.

As with the SCI individual, how the family reacts will greatly depend on their past coping mechanisms and how well the family is structured. A close-knit family with a well-defined communication system will fare much better than a family that is disorganized and has ill-defined coping skills.

PHYSICAL AND PSYCHOLOGICAL DATA

SUBJECTIVE

Patients often report that they don't know the exact date of the onset of the sore. Because they usually have not been inspecting their skin daily with a mirror, the first sign of a sore may be drainage noted on clothing or bedding from an already well-established sore. Many times, patients will admit to sitting in their wheelchairs for prolonged amounts of time or failing to turn properly while in bed. Other patients may blame wheelchair cushions or mattresses as being faulty or inferior and causing the sore. Some total-care patients will relate that their families or attendants have been negligent in their skin care or that the aide has deserted them, causing them to break down in their routines of self-care. Many patients will report a past history of sores and may even blame past surgeries for being ineffective and contributing to yet another sore. Most patients are well versed and can repeat methods of sore prevention. They are, however, equally proficient in explaining how such methods don't fit into their lifestyles (i.e., their job demands that they be up in the wheelchair long hours each day; they get bored staying in bed if they've developed reddened areas; it's too much trouble for the aide to get them out of bed for only one to hours hours a day; and so forth). Occasionally a patient may be unaware that he has a sore and will present to the clinic with a variety of complaints. If a patient presents complaints of increased spasticity, symptoms of autonomic dysreflexia, or a vague complaint that he isn't feeling "quite right," he should be examined for the possibility of a pressure sore.

Psychologically, the patient may express feelings of depression, lack of self-worth, an inability to cope with his injury and self-care, and may even voice suicidal ideation. He will, many times, voice his frustration and discouragement over the development of a sore. It must be remembered that assessment of these statements is just as critical as the statements concerning the physical aspects of the sore.

OBJECTIVE

Upon physical examination, pressure sores will most commonly be found on the SCI patient corresponding to the area where he spends the most time. If he is bedridden, sores will be found on the sacrum, greater trochanter, and heels. If in the wheelchair, the patient will develop coccyx and ischial sores (Ruge 1969). The sore must be classified according to its size, shape, depth, edges, floor, base, and drainage, if any. Observation must also be made of any dressing or treatment the patient has been applying to the sore, and the appearance of any foul odor. Surrounding tissues may appear reddened and inflamed and may feel "boggy" if the sore is undermined and filled with fluid. If the sore invades the muscle, there may be ectopic calcification or contractures (El torai 1977). Skin condition, in general, may be poor with evidence of other breakdown areas, such as poor hygiene, dryness, and decreased turgor. There may be extensive skin scarring if there is a past history of sores requiring surgical closure. Patients may appear rundown if anemic, and the skin and mucous membranes may appear pale. The patient who is prone to sores is often hypotensive. Clothing may be ill-fitting or rough; the cushion worn or defective; and the posture poor. Observation should be made during the history and physical exam as to whether the patients lift or shift their weight every 15 minutes. Oftentimes, this behavior will be absent. Objective clues to psychological status can be obtained from observing the patient's action. He may express his frustration and anger by grimacing, crying, wringing his hands, flailing his arms, or shouting. If self-abusive, he may strike himself. His effect may be inappropriate, and he may laugh or appear unaffected by the diagnosis. Whatever the case, these actions must be weighed carefully during the patient's assessment.

MANAGEMENT

DIAGNOSTIC PLAN

Depending on the findings of the physical examination and classification on the grading scale, workup may be deemed necessary as follows:

1. CBC/differential to rule out anemia or presence of infection
2. electrolyte panels to rule out electrolyte imbalance
3. serum protein to rule out hypoproteinemia
4. blood culture, if temperature of 102 degrees or greater, to rule out septicemia
5. C and S/gram stain of wound drainage to determine the presence of any infecting organisms.

For Grade IV and some Grade III patients, El torai (1977) additionally suggests:

1. X-ray of affected bones or joints to rule out any degenerative changes
2. a sinogram, if a sinus tract is involved, to determine if there is any communication with bones, joints, or body cavities
3. a possible bone scan to rule out osteomylitis or ectopic calcification
4. tissue stress studies to determine extent of tissue involvement.

THERAPEUTIC PLAN

Treatment will vary from patient to patient and from sore to sore. A review of the literature indicates that many different methods have been employed in the treatment of sores. No matter what the therapeutic plan, it should strive to attain the following goals (Easterby 1977):

1. relieve the pressure
2. clear infection
3. remove necrosi
4. affect the earliest rehabilitation, mobilization, and discharge.

From a prognostic and treatment approach, Grade I and II pressure sores are considered similar, as are Grade III and IV. Therefore, the management plan will be divided into two parts. Regardless of the anatomic location of the pressure sore, the basic management is the same.

Treatment for Grade I or II Pressure Sore

1. The hallmark of treatment for this diagnosis is relief of pressure on the area of tissue insult. This can be accomplished in bed by use of the prone position. If the patient cannot tolerate this position, then the side-back-side positions are used. Always try to avoid using the position where the pressure sore has occurred. If this position must be used, the bridging technique is used in positioning. This technique utilizes pillows positioned above and below the area of insult so when the patient is turned onto the area, it is free of any pressure. It is important to roll or lift the patient and not drag him so that he does not suffer any shear-stress damage to his skin. If the sore is not on the ischii, the patient is allowed to sit up in the wheelchair, but he must have a cushion in the chair to alleviate pressure. The

goal of a proper cushion fit is to have a pressure of less than 35 mmHg under bony prominences. This cushion needs to be reevaluated and changed as it wears out, or if the patient should develop reddened areas. Remember, pressure-relieving devices cannot be substituted for proper turning and lifting. Never use plaster casts, sandbags, or hard pillows for immobilizing or positioning the SCI patient.

2. The area needs to be cleaned twice daily, or more often if the patient is incontinent, to control bacterial contamination. Soap is not recommended because its alkalines make the horny layers of the skin swell and damage the epidermis with their keralolytic and caustic effect. There is much controversy regarding the type of solution or agent to be used in this process. A review of the historical literature reveals the following have been used: poultices of carrots and turnips, bread and charcoal, proteolytic enzymes, cortisone, vitamin preparations, dried blood plasma, gold leaf, alcohol, chlorophyll, sugar, and brine baths. There is no conclusive evidence that one modality is superior to another. Probably used the most frequently at the present time is Betadine Solution and hydrogen peroxide for cleansing, followed by covering of the area with a dry sterile dressing and nonallergic tape. It may be left open to air if there are any signs of maceration. The dressing should not be stretches under tension, as this would cause excoriation of skin margins.

3. A high-protein diet with vitamin C supplement is encouraged, since protein is needed for tissue growth. Patient's food preferences need to be assessed and incorporated into the dietary planning. If there is a loss of appetite, small, frequent feedings are in order.

4. Assurance, counseling and emotional support need to be provided.

5. If pressure is relieved and a high-protein diet is maintained, the reactive process of Grade I and II pressure sores resolve in 5 to 14 days.

6. Patient and family education should include information about the following:

a. The importance of the prevention of pressure sores needs to be stressed, because it is easier and less costly than the treatment and care necessary for healing the insult.

b. Ischial pressure relief every one hour for 60 seconds while sitting in a wheelchair needs to be demonstrated. Patient needs to be encouraged to become more aware of actively incorporating this into his daily regime.

c. When the patient remains in bed for a period of time, he should be turned every two hours or he should be proned (turned to lie on his stomach) on a sheepskin.

d. Inspect skin in nonsensate areas morning and night with a mirror. If any areas of erythema are noted, patient should be taught to stay off these areas to prevent pressure areas.

e. Teach methods of fecal and urinary continence to prevent skin maceration.

f. Explain the importance of a cushion pressure evaluation every six months or sooner if erythematous areas appear on the ischii. Most high-density foam cushions need to be replaced every six months. Air rings or donuts should be avoided since they reduce the blood supply to the area.

g. Importance of daily hygiene and proper drying of skin, especially in areas covered by clothing, should be stressed.

Treatment for Grade III and IV Pressure Sores in Addition to the Treatment Outline for Grades I and II Sores

1. Treatment of any anemia, if present, by iron supplementation and vitamins, or transfusion if anemia is profound. A hemoglobin greater than 12.5 gms is necessary for proper skin healing (Guthrie 1969).

2. Appropriate systemic antibiotics are give either P.O. or IV if the patient has signs of septicemia. Since systemic antibiotics do not reach the pressure sore because of poor tissue perfusion in the ulcerated area, their use is usually reserved for septic patients.

3. High-protein diet alone will not balance what is being lost by drainage from the pressure sore, so hyperalimentation feedings are usually given to restore nutritional status. Nonvirilesing androgens are sometimes given because they act as protein-sparing agents. Electrolyte replacement is included in the hyperalimentation formula. A few patients may require parenteral hyperalimentation if their intestine does not tolerate the high-protein formula.

4. All necrotic tissue must be removed. Debridement of small areas of necrotic tissue can be accomplished by wet to dry dressings. Use of enzymatic agents (i.e., collagenase, debrison, etc.) may help debride superficial sores. Surgical excision is required for large areas of necrotic tissue and to evacuate abscess formation.

5. In presence of osteomyelitis, hyperbaric oxygen, as well as surgical drainage, may promote healing.

6. Laser therapy is the use of a narrow beam of light of concentrated high energies. This is being used experimentally with treatment of pressure areas.

7. After all conservative measures have been instituted and the wound is pink and lined with granulation tissue, surgical closure is advocated to cut down on time spent in the hospital (El torai 1977). Flap closure gives durable full thickness repair which is important over bony prominences. Wound edges that are approximated in a linear fashion may cause undue skin tension and not give maximum protection. After the plastic repair has been done, the patient must remain flat in a position that does not produce

pressure on the surgical site for four to eight weeks to allow healing. Post-op complications to be watched for are infection, wound separation, sloughing, or failure of a graft to take. When the bed rest period is over, the patient starts sitting in a wheelchair on a cushion with reduced pressure. This sitting program is for one half-hour the first day, then increased by half-hour increments on subsequent days. If erythema is not present, the goal is maximum sitting tolerance of six to eight hours. Be sure that when the patient is turned in bed he is lifted from position to position and not dragged, as this will cause shearing of skin with surfaces below. Time spent in the hospital for Grades III and IV pressure sores is three to six months when plastic repair is done. When the wound is healed by secondary intention, the time is increased to nine to twelve months. It is important during the long convalescence to provide psychological counseling and diversional activities.

PATIENT EDUCATION

In addition to what is taught for Grades I and II pressure sores, education includes information regarding the following:

1.   The site of repair will not resist pressure as well as previously intact skin.

2.   If the area has healed by secondary intention and not surgery, the patient must recognize that the scar is thin, avascular, friable and adherent to the structures beneath it. Therefore, it is easier to break down with minimum pressure.

3.   Heat or ultraviolet lamps must not be used, as they cause burns.

4.   There is a need to become conscious of the hourly ritual of position change necessary for pressure relief.

5.   Understanding the importance of seeking medical attention at earliest signs of recurrence of pressure sores is necessary.

6.   Dressing changes or other care of the wound will promote self-care status to the greatest possible extent. Tasks should be geared so that the patient can have mastery over his environment. This will enhance self-esteem.

8

Respiratory Complications

MARY JANE CALLAHAN and WILMA TAYLOR

Maintaining respiratory function and preventing respiratory embarrassment are immediate and life-long concerns of the spinal cord–injured patient (Sutton 1973). In the immediate or acute stage following the injury, the extent of paralysis will determine the necessary respiratory interventions to maintain life. While the higher-level spinal injuries involve more of the respiratory musculature, many of the lower-level spinal injuries may involve rib or sternum fractures that also readily compromise the respiratory system (Guttman 1976).

Those who survive the acute and the immediate post-acute stages will need to concern themselves with good respiratory health. As with any chronically disabled person, the limited activity, decreased physical strength, and susceptibility to infection can cause respiratory illness (Wade 1977).

INCIDENCE, EPIDEMIOLOGY, AND PATHOPHYSIOLOGY

The National Spinal Cord Injury Data Research reports that in a group of 182 quadriplegics, 22 deaths occurred, and in all cases the primary cause of death was cardio-pulmonary complications. Fifty percent of the patients with spinal cord injuries have significant hypoxemia. Some have oxygen tension of less than 60 mmHg without prior lung disease (Petty 1974). The normal physiology of the respiratory system is dependent on the contraction of respiratory musculature. The muscles are also utilized for the processes of vocalizing, coughing, sneezing, sighing, and straining. These functions should appropriately take place without interfering with normal respiration (Montero and Feldman 1965).

The primary muscle of respiration is the diaphragm. This dome-shaped muscle is located between the thorax and abdomen and is enervated by the two phrenic nerves, which arise from the third and fourth cervical nerves

(Wade 1971). The diaphragm controls 60 percent of the inspiration. The external intercostals and scaleni muscles control the other 40 percent. When these muscles are weakened or unable to function, the sterno-cleidomastoids, trapezeus, serratus anterior and even the platysma will assist in the inspiratory process (Montero and Feldman 1965).

Expiration, in which the lung returns to its resting state, is normally passive. But when more tidal volume is needed for increased activities, the intercostals as well as the abdominal muscles will be used to increase expiratory effort (Montero and Feldman 1965).

Injuries or disease of the spinal cord result in varying degrees of paralysis. In cord injuries involving the first to the seventh cervical vertebrae, there will be paralysis of the upper and lower limbs (quadriplegia). The thoracic spinal cord injuries usually arise from fractures or displacement of the eleventh and twelfth vertebrae. This level of injury frequently involves the first lumbar as well and will produce paralysis of the various corresponding segmental levels that will also include the lower limbs (paraplegia) (Guttman 1976).

Almost all quadriplegics who survive have sustained an injury no higher than the third cervical level, and they will have pulmonary insufficiency. There is flaccid paralysis of the intercostal and abdominal muscles in the acute stages, which results in two-thirds normal inspiratory capability and almost no expiratory volume. This almost completely abolishes forced expiration and productive coughing. There is also impairment in the mechanics of swallowing, which greatly increases the probability of aspiration.

Injury resulting in paraplegia frequently is the result of either a falling object striking the victim while he is a flexed, crouched position or of a vehicular accident. These patients frequently have accompanying fractures of the rib and sternum resulting in hemo- or pneumothorax (Carini Owens 1974). Further contributing to the problem during the acute period in many patients is bowel paralysis, with an acutely dilated stomach that will inhibit thoracic expansion and increase respiratory distress (Montero and Feldman 1965). Pulmonary embolism is a major complication following severe injuries. The combination of enforced bed rest, muscular paralysis, and vasomotor paralysis increases venous stasis. The incidence of venous thrombosis in spinal cord injury is approximately 60 percent and in a number of patients results in pulmonary embolism (Haas 1965).

Another problem in the pathophysiology of the cardio-pulmonary system is interruption of the sympathetic enervation and control of the vago vagal reflex. As a result, most quadriplegics are bradycardic. Low arterial PO2 may produce a cardiac block or arrest (Wade 1977). Pneumonia is another result of pathological changes in the respiratory process, because these often result in decreased ability of the diaphragm, intercostals, and abdominal muscles to clear lung secretion. Retained secretions lead to atelectasis because they provide a medium for bacterial growth and hypostatic pneumonia. Repeated infections result in chronic infections, and eventually quadriplegia may result in chronic organic pulmonary disease. The patient who already has pulmonary organic disease when injured has even more problems. To maintain adequate PO2 levels, these patients may need continuous mechanical ventilation for several months (Carter 1979).

PSYCHOSOCIAL COMPONENTS

The spinal cord–injured patient spends much of the time during the post-injury period learning to live with the new physical disabilities and impaired respiration. Essential to successful rehabilitation is the ability to become integrated into society as a disabled person (Trieschmann 1980). The important factor will be how the patient views himself with his disability, for it will affect his interactions with the people around him. His behavior can evoke pity, anger, rejection, or a reserved tolerance. These reactions may not be helpful to his resocialization. His friends will see him as different from his pre-injury state, and this could lead to social isolation, particularly if he has not been prepared to cope with this aspect of his rehabilitation. The extent to which the patient is able to overcome his social discomfort will also depend on his pre-injury personality and how he perceived disabled people (Gunther 1976).

Rotter (1969) hypothesized that some people believe in an external locus of control that dictates the happenings in their lives. They see forces as being beyond their personal dictates and resulting from chance or luck. Other persons believe in an internal locus of control and see rewards and punishments as the result of their own actions. Persons with an external orientation believe that what happens to them is not elated to their actions, and so they have low expectations of their activities. Internal locus of control people are more apt to see outcomes as a result of their own efforts. Therefore the goals that the rehabilitation team subscribes will probably be more meaningful to the patient with an internal locus of control. When locus of control orientation is considered in providing supportive care and encouraging pa ients to be involved in their area, the patient may benefit (Gunther 1969).

The family members are almost as greatly affected by the spinal injury and its accompanying respiratory complications as the patient. They need to understand and accept the injury as a reality. Because of the family's importance to the patient, their attitudes toward him will be most significant. While attempting to be supportive of the patient, their own fears may affect and disrupt the patient's coping attempts (Kahn 1969). The family should be considered a part of the rehabilitation team. They should visit the therapy sessions, where they can view the procedures and ask questions. From the very beginning they should be made aware of the patient's progress and be given complete explanations. Seeing the patient in the intensive care unit, depending on a respirator for breathing, may have a profound effect on close family members. While being given information they also should be allowed the opportunity to express their feelings (Kahn 1969).

The patient's physical needs may be more of a burden than the family can manage. A young mother, for instance, faced with providing financial support and caring for young children, may be overwhelmed. She may be bitter about the circumstances that she is now confronted with and experience guilt because of her feelings. She may also have difficulty expressing her feelings to her family. Clinical studies suggest that those marriages that were troubled before injury will be stressed further by the injury. Similarly, the pre-injury state of a marriage will probably affect the state of the post-injury environment of the couple (Trieschmann 1980).

PHYSICAL AND PSYCHOLOGICAL COMPONENTS

SUBJECTIVE DATA

Many patients report being aware of their paralysis immediately upon injury. But since the spinal cord injury usually occurs in a traumatic incident, victims may be unconscious and completely dependent on their rescuers to recognize their emergency needs.

During the first part of their hospitalization patients may not be able to comprehend the full extent of their injuries. They are in a strange environment, surrounded by complex equipment, with formal physical capabilities to help them adapt and cope (Pierce and Nickel 1977).

Cervical-injured patients will be disturbed with their altered breathing. They will become increasingly apprehensive and frightened when left alone. They cannot move and do not have enough breath to yell. The newly injured may not be able to operate even the most sensitive call light that responds to minimal pressure. If they have had a tracheotomy, their anxiety will be increased, since they cannot speak or question what is happening (Kirilloff and Maszkiewcz 1979). Because of the difficulties in communication, the practitioner must be sensitive to observable clues that assist in the recognition of the patient's needs.

Psychologically, the patient may have feelings of unreality, that he is not actually in an injured situation. There will be a loss of night-and-day reality. In the intensive care units the lights are on all the time. Stress and pain as well as hypoxia will interfere with logical thought and will distort what is happening and what is being done. The patient must accept what has happened and deal with the trauma of an altered image before being able to adapt to a new lifestyle. Smithermann (1981) sees severe injury as causing the loss of self-esteem. Self-esteem is seen as a measure of one's own personal worth. Most people equate self-worth with being physically strong and capable.

We establish our self-images fairly early in our lives, but we are constantly refining and redefining ourselves according to our life's experiences and changing roles. The spinal cord injury will affect the self-image concept, and patients will be forced to see themselves in an unexpected role that will probably be permanent. Their feeling of being different may prevent them from recognizing any value in life or may overwhelm them to the point of withdrawal (Vash 1978). It is difficult to separate the psychological from the physical dynamics because the patient's frame of mind will affect the physical process. The altered physiological state that has occurred because of the cord injury affects all of the body systems. Anxiety increases respiratory needs. The depressed vasomotor activity increases pooling of blood, and cardiac output is decreased. The total bodily effort to maintain homeostasis is exhausting. The patient will complain of fatigue. It is important at this stage to allow dependency until the patient can adjust to the physiological changes that are being undergone (Smithermann 1981).

The extent of the hardship a disability will impose depends upon the degree of disability, the task at hand, and the patient's level of adjustment. Some tasks will reveal greater disability than others. A quadriplegic sitting in a chair talking to his son does not seem as disabled as a quadriplegic trying to bathe his son. When patients are able to accept what has happened to their·bodies as something that must be dealt with, they are preparing to recognize themselves as they are (Vash 1978).

OBJECTIVE DATA

As already stated, respiratory failure is most frequent in the immediate post-injury period when the third or fourth cervical segments are involved. High thoracic injuries may also have respiratory impairment, and lower-spine injuries can also spread up the cord and involve the respiratory muscles. Paralysis of the intercostals decreases lung expansion. The sympathetic pathways from the hypothalamus to the thoracic cord level are interrupted, and respiratory stimulation is impaired (Sutton 1973). The objective data on admission will include a rapid assessment of respiratory involvement. It is important to observe if the chest and accessory muscles are moving or if there is only abdominal breathing. Auscultation of the chest will reveal the presence or absence of breath sounds. It is important to note if there are signs of vomitus. Chest X-rays, routine laboratory studies, measurement of vital capacity, and evaluation of arterial blood gases should be done. The patient's workup should include the history, a physical and neurological examination, and also any past history of smoking, pulmonary disease, or allergies (Carter 1979). Atelectasis *and* infection are an ever-present problem, and culture and sensitivity of the sputum should be obtained.

The psychological data should include the behavior responses that are evident in the patient. The normal range of responses to be expected at various times during the hospitalization include anxiety, denial, grief, and depression. Changes of moods will be evident with fluctuations from day to day (Smithermann 1981). Much of our behavior responses are learned behaviors and therefore will vary according to past experiences. A patient's inability to sleep, eat, and cooperate with appropriate therapy schedules may be indicative of problems. Gastrointestinal upsets when no physical cause can be determined may be a reaction to stress. If feelings of anxiety and helplessness overwhelm the patient, the reaction may be anger. This prevents interaction with other people. When anger is evident, the practitioner may help the patient express this anger appropriately and thus prevent depression, which is a frequent consequence (Trieschmann 1980).

MANAGEMENT

DIAGNOSTIC PLAN

In the immediate stage following injury, the patient with trauma to the cervical area is given top priority in treatment because of the neuroanatomical and physiological effects on the respiratory system. An open airway must be established with the proper ventilatory assistance. A tracheotomy may be necessary for the quadriplegic who has a cervical four and five injury with apnea (Carini and Owens 1978). In a comatose patient who is breathing, the observance of upper-chest movement greater than lower-chest movement is diagnostic of spinal cord injury. Carter (1979) recommends measuring vital capacity at least once every eight hours. Frequent blood gases and pH determinations are needed to determine adequacy of ventilation. The patient who has extensive wounds with possible internal injuries will need to be typed and cross-matched for blood replacement in the event of surgery. A rapid assessment is done to determine the neurological involvement by testing for the deep tendon reflexes. Chest X-rays are done to detect atelectasis as well as possible rib or sternum fractures. Films are ordered of the skull and spine to determine the level of injury and whether there is need for immediate surgery to stabilize the spine (Guttman 1976).

Since these patients may be unable to swallow or cough effectively, the staff must be alert to the possibility of pulmonary aspiration, infection, and pneumothorax that would further aggravate hypoventilation (Carini and Owens 1974). A one-sided diaphragmatic paralysis is suspected in an adult quadriplegic whose vital capacity is less than 1000 cc. A double-exposure X-ray showing both inspiration and expiration will confirm the diagnosis.

Because of stress due to the injury or following surgery, a gastric ulcer may develop and possibly bleed or perforate. This can cause abdominal distention and elevate the diaphragm into the thorax and decrease vital capacity. Hepatic dullness is generally absent with perforated stress ulcers and present with acute gastric dilation or ileus (Rothman and Simeone 1974).

Another problem is pulmonary embolism. The quadriplegic does not complain of pain but usually complains of sudden shortness of breath. The vital capacity will be adequate, but there will be a decrease in the PO2 (Larrabee 1977).

THERAPEUTIC PLAN

A therapeutic plan should be in readiness for the patient with a cervical injury. The possibility of respiratory embarrassment should be anticipated, as the injury may affect the phrenic nerves (McCormick 1974). Equipment on hand should include oxygen as well as a tracheotomy tray and suctioning equipment. Some patients may need the assistance of a ventilator. If the patient is able to breathe independently, oxygen therapy may be sufficient (Larrabee 1977).

The patient with a cervical injury will need careful observation, particularly if he has a tracheotomy. Frequent tracheobronchial suctioning and sterile technique should be used to prevent introducing bacteria into the respiratory tract. The patient's oxygen reserve is limited, so care must be taken not to deplete it further when suctioning. This can be done by limiting the suctioning to 8 to 10 second intervals (Wade 1977). To prevent drying of mucous membranes and formation of hard mucous plugs, humidified air/oxygen is used during the acute period. If congestion is noted, a bronchodilator and mucolytic drugs are added to a nebulizer. To promote coughing, clapping or vibratory stimulation should be done (Wade 1977).

Gastric distention is relieved with the insertion of a nasogastric tube. This decreases thoracic pressure, helps to prevent vomiting, and thereby decreases the possibility of aspiration (Rothman and Simeone 1974).

Edema of the cord is treated with large doses of steroids. Antacids (magnesium and aluminum hydroxide) may be given by nasogastric tube or orally to prevent the stress ulcer secondary to high-dose steroid therapy

(Larrabee 1977). Cimetidine is indicated for patients with high gastric acid secretion.

Nasal congestion is a problem for quadriplegics. The problem is present when the patient is in the supine position and cannot tolerate the prone position at all. The frequent use of antihistamines produces a rebound effect and needs to be discouraged.

The long-term therapeutic plan calls for maintaining vital capacity by strengthening respiratory musculature. The patient should stop smoking. The physical therapist will develop a program of exercises, and the patient should be encouraged to carry it out routinely after discharge.

Phrenic Nerve Stimulation

The spinal cord–injured patient with an injury proximal to C-3, C-4, or C-5 segments may be a candidate for a phrenic pacemaker (Carter 1979). The proximal injury produces an upper motor neuron lesion with an intact lower motor unit. The pacemaker converts radio frequency signals into small, continuous electrical impulses that stimulate the phrenic nerve. Stimulation of the intact nerve triggers the diaphragm to descend and allows inspiration to take place. If the spinal cord injury occurs at the C-3, C-4 or C-5 segments of the spinal cord, the results are poor due to damage to the anterior horn cells resulting in peripheral degeneration of the lower motor neurons. This condition causes flaccid paralysis of the diaphragm. Stimulation of the phrenic nerve in this situation will not affect diaphragm contraction (Vanderlinden et al. 1974). A person who has suffered an immediate, complete quadriplegia at the C-1 or C-2 level and is dependent on a mechanical respirator is a candidate for electrophrenic respiration implant surgery. The intact lower motor neurons in the phrenic nerve may be confirmed by surface stimulation under fluroscopy exam over the phrenic nerve at the base of the neck, causing diaphragm contraction.

The person who suffers an immediate quadriplegia at the C-4 or C-5 level, who is initially breathing voluntarily and subsequently develops paralysis of the diaphragm and becomes respirator-dependent, is not a candidate for this technique due to lower motor neuron damage. It also cannot be successfully used when there is impaired pulmonary and diaphragmatic function, partial destruction or interruption of the phrenic nerve, or any disease that affects nerve conduction such as a tumor, muscular disease, diabetic neuropathy, or multiple sclerosis. Failure to significantly improve the arterial PCO_2 and PO_2 is an indication that diaphragm pacing will not be effective.

Knowledge of the operation of the pacer is helpful in assessing effectiveness and trouble-shooting. Each inspiration is initiated by a train of about forty gradually increasing electrical pulses, which produce a smooth contracting of the diaphragm, closely resembling normal breathing. An external battery-powered transmitter develops a coded radio frequency signal that is radiated across the intact skin from a loop transmitting antenna to an implanted passive radio receiver. The receiver demodulates the signal and delivers the resulting direct current pulses to a bipolar electrode placed on the phrenic nerve. The inspiration time, the respiration rate, and the amplitude of the stimulating pulse are controlled from the external transmitter.

The implant operation can be done under local anesthetic and can be accomplished in one or two stages. Both phrenic nerves can be paced in one procedure, but it is more often accomplished in two stages about four months apart. The quadriplegic patient who has been apneic for a long period will require six to eight weeks of gradually increasing periods of stimulation before the phrenic nerve can be electrically excited for 10 to 12 hours without diaphragm fatigue. When not on the stimulator, his respirations require the same assistance as before implantation. During the period of diaphragm conditioning, the tidal volume is used as a guide to increase pacing time. When post-stimulation volume measures at least 75 percent of prestimulation volume, the pacing period can be extended. The goal is to achieve stimulation of the left phrenic nerve for 12 hours, and then the right phrenic nerve for 12 hours while the alternate nerve is resting. In some patients the transmission has been combined to provide alternate stimulation. Possible complications include:

1. injury to the phrenic nerve by the pacemaker cuff or by reduction or nerve blood supply due to edema or technique
2. diaphragm fatigue related to prolonged period of nerve stimulation
3. implant site infection
4. pacemaker failure
5. upper airway obstruction.

Bantam Respirator

Another breathing aid is the Bantam positive pressure respirator. The Bantam provides mechanical inspiratory assistance, delivering room air. This respirator allows the patient to get out of bed and to be mobile. The patient can use the respirator for four or five hours before the battery will need to be recharged (Benvenuti 1979).

PATIENT EDUCATION

Patients should be informed of their condition and progress throughout their hospital stay. At first, information is kept simple and serves to alleviate anxiety. Patients will have many concerns about what is happening to them. Respiratory insufficiency is an early complication, and patients will be concerned about their altered breathing. They may not put these concerns into words; they may not, in fact, be able to speak. The practitioner should offer explanations when she senses the patient's concern or anxiety when she performs suctioning or ventilatory treatments. Offering support and help will reassure the patient that people are concerned and ready to help (Smithermann 1981).

The physical therapist will teach patients to stretch their lungs by a controlled inhalation of air. The patient should be taught the use of the incentive spirometer. This exercise will also promote productive coughing (Larrabee 1977). The patient's education should include an explanation of why his secretions pool and how this can result in pulmonary infection. The patient and family should be instructed in the manner of pulmonary toileting with postural drainage, clapping, and assisted coughing (Wade 1976). The patient should avoid people with cold symptoms. Both paraplegics and quadriplegics should be encouraged to have yearly flu shots. Pneumonia will always be a potential problem to quadriplegics and needs to be treated promptly (Sutton 1973). Maintaining adequate respiratory function requires the cooperation of the patient and the entire rehabilitation team.

9

Sexual Dysfunction

MARY ANN CARROLL, TERESA OWEN TEMPKIN,
and WILLIAM WORTH

There are estimated to be some 120,000 people with spinal cord injury in the United States today. Eighty percent of the injured persons are male. As women have become more physically active, they have also become more prone to spinal cord injury. Thus the percentage of women with new injuries each year seems to be increasing. The law of spinal cord states that if there is an injury to the spinal cord, at the level of the injury there will never be a return of reflex activity. The law also states that once spinal shock is over there will be a return of reflex activity below the level of the injury (Comarr 1977b). Damage to the cord at the level of injury will involve pathways from the brain to the spinal cord—the upper motor neurons (UMN)—with reflex activity. Also involved by damage to the cord at the level of injury will be the pathways from the cord to the muscles—the lower motor neurons (LMN)—with no reflex activity. If these injuries are incomplete, psychogenic erections may occur in the male and psychogenic excitement in the female. The extent of the sexual dysfunction is difficult to predict since the amount of neurological damage varies in each individual.

NEUROPHYSIOLOGY AND PATHOPHYSIOLOGY OF SEXUAL FUNCTION IN THE MALE

Normal sexual function in males is a complicated physiologic process involving all three components of the peripheral nervous system: the parasympathetic, the sympathetic, and the somatic systems. A brief explanation of the neurophysiology involved in the sex act will help clarify the processes involved in a spinal cord injury. The physical aspect of male sexual function can be viewed as involving four phenomena: erection, emission, ejaculation, and orgasm. The descriptions of the phenomena that follows are excerpted from Rabin (1980).

1. *Erection.*   There are two types, reflexogenic and psychogenic.
   Reflex erections may be initiated by stimulation from the pelvic region, the glans penis, urethra, prostate gland or a full bladder. The sensory impulses are carried from these parts by the dorsal nerve of the penis to the pudendal nerve and on to the sacral 2 to 4 segments (S 2–4). Impulses to these sacral segments may also come from the pelvic nerve. From these sacral segments, the impulses go back by motor impulses through two nerves. The impulse through the pelvic nerve causes the arteries in the corpora cavernose of the penis to dilate and become engorged with blood. This stiffens the penis so it is capable of intromission. The impulse through the pudendal nerve causes the bulbo and ischiocavernosus muscles to contract, decreasing the blood outflow in the veins from the penis. This coordinated action of the pelvic and pudendal nerves maintains the erection. This reflex involves only the parasympathetic nervous system. If the physical stimulation does not continue, the erection will be lost. Reflexogenic erections occur independent of the brain. This is true for the able bodied male as well as the SCI male. If the break in the spinal cord is above the sacral segments, reflex erections will occur even though there is no connection between the genital area and the brain.

   The psychogenic type of erection involves stimuli that are processed through the cortical brain centers. These may be a combination of visual, auditory, or olfactory stimuli, or that of previous learning. The impulses come from the brain down the cord, where they leave somewhere between the T-9 and L-2 segments. From here the impulses reach the pelvic area via the presacral nerves and hypogastric complexes. Psychogenic erections are achieved through the sympathetic nervous system. Generally, the psychogenic and reflexogenic components of erection complement each other. In a spinal cord–injured male, however, these influences may work independently of each other or may even inhibit each other.

2. *Emission.*   Emission is a function of the sympathetic nervous system. The sensory impulses, originating from stimulation in the pelvic area, travel along the internal pudendal nerve to the spinal cord. Motor impulses then leave the spinal cord somewhere between T–11 and L 1–3 segments and travel through the presacral nerves to the hypogastric plexus. From there the impulses reach the epididymis, the vas deferens, and the prostate gland. The smooth muscles of these structures then contract, sending the sperm, with accompanying secretions, into the posterior urethra where emission stays before ejaculation. This lasts only a few seconds and is the first part of the subjective feeling of orgasm.

3. *Ejaculation.*   The emission of semen into the posterior urethra is the trigger impulse which sends motor impulses through the pudendal nerve to sacral segments 2–4 and then back to the perineal muscles. Impulses from S 2–4 also reach higher cortical levels, with impulses sent back down through T-9 to L-3 levels. These impulses cause the urethra containing the semen to contract. The contraction propels the semen from the urethra. At the same time, the internal sphincter is contracted by the sympathetic nerves, preventing retrograde ejaculation; and the external sphincter is enervated by the pudendal nerve, which opens to permit the semen to escape.

4. *Orgasm.*   Neurophysical explanations of the orgasm involve essentially the same process as those for emission and ejaculation. The impulses of ejaculation reach the brain, bringing awareness of the sensations. The importance of the neural connections is that the sensations are being interpreted by the brain and are not necessarily fully dependent on genital sensation. This fact allows all sorts of influences to enhance or inhibit the feel or orgasm. During orgasm various parts of the body may be involved and undergo changes in terms of tension and relaxation. Generally, there is a combination of genital and total body response [Rabin 1980].

The impotent male is defined as being completely, or partially, unable to initiate, sustain, or successfully conclude the act of intercourse (Wood and Rose 1978). Impotence is classified as psychogenic or organic in origin. The spinal cord injury patient has an organic basis for impotence, although the impotence almost always has strong psychological ramifications.

Organic impotence is defined as the loss of ability to obtain and/or maintain a functional erection, due to the interruption of certain physiological processes (Small, Carrion, and Gordon 1975). Organic impotence can be caused by:

1. trauma
    a. spinal cord injury
    b. pelvic fracture
2. postoperative condition after
    a. prostatectomy
    b. cystectomy
    c. external sphincterotomy
    d. abdominal perineal resection
3. vascular disease
    a. arteriosclerosis
    b. priapism

4. neurologic disease
   a. peripheral neuropathy
   b. multiple sclerosis
5. endocrine and metabolic disease
   a. diabetes
   b. hypogonadism
   c. renal failure
6. medications
   a. exogenous estrogen
   b. parasympatholytics
   c. narcotics, e.g., morphine, heroin (Small, Carrion, and Gordon 1975).

The process involved in normal male sexual function must be kept in mind when considering the effects of a spinal cord injury on sexual capabilities. Immediately after a spinal cord injury, the individual enters a period called spinal shock in which there is no sensation or motor activity below the level of injury. This state has been reported to last from days to months, and an accurate assessment of the patient's sexual functioning cannot be made until the spinal shock resolves. This does not mean that sexual function should not be discussed with the patient, but the complete picture is not known yet, and so cannot be shared with him.

When the individual begins to come out of spinal shock, a careful detailed history and physical exam should be done by the practitioner, and any and all changes noted. Most important is the neurological exam. Without a complete examination, the injured person's sexual potential cannot be precisely ascertained.

The sexual diagnosis is dependent on whether reflex activity is or is not present through the S2–S4 segments of the spinal cord via the internal pudendal nerve. If reflex activity is present through the pudendal nerve, it will usually, although not always, be present also through the pelvic nerve (nervi erigentes), which is the parasympahetic element involved in sexual function. The presence or absence of reflex activity through S2–S4 segments is ascertained by performing a rectal examination. This is to ascertain the presence or absence of:

1. external anal sphincter tone
2. bulbocavernosus reflex
3. pinprick sensation in the saddle area bilaterally (Cressy and Comarr 1981).

The presence of tone in the external rectal sphincter, a positive bulbocavernosus reflex, or both, indicates that the patient has an upper motor neuron lesion (UMN-reflex) and is capable of reflexogenic erection. The absence of external rectal sphincter tone, an absent bulbocavernosus reflex, or both, indicates that the patient has a lower motor neuron (LMN-areflexic) involvement and is capable of areflexic sexual function (Comarr 1975). These classifications indicate only the presence or absence of somatic reflex activity through the sacral segments and autonomic reflex activity by inference. It must then be ascertained if sensation is reaching the brain through the sacral segments and whether the brain can send volitional messages down and through the sacral segments to reach the target striated muscles. The former is tested by using a pin (or paper clip) to the penis, scrotum, perianal area, S1 segment of the foot and S2 segment of the posterior thigh dermatomes bilaterally. The latter is tested by asking the patient to volitionally contract, on command, the external anal sphincter (Cressy and Comarr 1981).

There are four types of lesions:

1. *Reflex complete (UMN).* Reflex activity is present through S2–S4 segments. Sensation in the penis, scrotum and perianal dermatomes and volitional control of the external anal sphincter are not present.
2. *Reflex incomplete (UMN).* Reflex activity is present through the S2–S4 segments. Sensation is present and volitional control is absent or vice versa. Partial sensation is present (pinprick or light touch) and/or partial or no volitional control of the external sphincter is present.
3. *Areflexic complete (LMN).* Reflex activity is absent through S2–S4 segments. Sensation in the penis, scrotum and perianal dermatomes and volitional control of the external anal sphincter are not present.
4. *Areflexic incomplete (LMN).* Reflex activity is absent through S2–S4 segments. Sensation is present and volitional control is absent or vice versa. Partial sensation is present and/or partial or no volitional control of the external sphincter is present.

Using this classification, the predicted expectations of sexual function among SCI males is reported as follows:

Reflex complete:

- Approximately 90 percent or more in this group can be expected to have reflexogenic erections.
- About 70 percent or less of the 90 percent will be able to have successful coitus.
- About 10 percent or less will not have erections of any type.
- The vast majority will not be able to ejaculate or have orgasm.

Reflex incomplete:

- Approximately 98 percent in this group are able to attain erections of one type of another.
- About 83 percent will have successful coitus.

- About 45 percent can be expected to have psychogenic erections.
- Of those patients who can have successful coitus, about 36 percent have been able to ejaculate. If, at times, psychogenic erections cannot be attained by those who usually can, reflexogenic erections can usually be attained.

Areflexic complete:

- The majority of these patients cannot have erections satisfactory for coitus.
- About 27 percent to 40 percent can have psychogenic erections.
- The success rate of those who attempt coitus ranges from 24 percent to 50 percent.
- Those who can ejaculate range from 19 percent to 35 percent.

Areflexic incomplete:

- 83 percent of this group have psychogenic erections.
- Of those that attempt coitus, 75 percent are successful, and 56 percent are able to ejaculate and have orgasm.

Siring of children:

- Of 287 patients with reflex complete lesions, 1 percent sired children.
- Of 123 patients with reflex incomplete lesions, 6 percent sired children.
- Of 109 patients with areflexic complete lesions, 5.6 percent sired children.
- Of 10 patients with areflexic incomplete lesions, 10 percent sired children (Cressey and Comarr 1981).

As the statistics show, fertility after a spinal cord injury is very low. There can be several reasons for this. The first is the inability of some SCI males to ejaculate. Another cause is retrograde ejaculation into the bladder. A third reason is testicular atrophy, which can happen as early as three or four months after the injury. The changes in heat regulatory mechanisms seem to have an influence on the atrophy process (Sandowski 1976). Testicular atrophy occurs with the loss of sympathetic enervation of the testicles and the resulting loss of intrascrotal temperature regulation; a cooler environment than that of the abdomen is necessary for spermatogenesis.

Sex can have various meanings to different people. Sex can be an activity culminating in orgasm, a method of procreation, a way of building self-esteem, a way of manipulating and controlling others, or an expression of tenderness, concern, and love. In many studies done with spinal cord–injured patients, it was found that the majority had some degree of genital function and that the need for sexual gratification, however perceived, remained a very important issue. Love (including sexual expression) is one of the strongest human emotions. It is important to remember that physical disability does not diminish an individual's need for love and affection. Spinal cord injury is a devastating experience for any active, independent individual, and it produces severe ramifications involving all aspects of one's biological, social and psychological mechanisms in attempting to cope with it (Crigler 1974).

With the loss of his sensation and control over bodily functions and movements, the individual feels stripped of his sexual identity, his body integrity, and his very purpose in life. The usual reaction to traumatic spinal cord injury is temporary depression related to the disability and the accompanying lowered self-esteem. The hope for complete recovery after a spinal cord injury is usually strong, and most patients employ some form of denial as a psychological defense against the realization that a profound and permanent injury has occurred. The total effect of spinal cord injury upon the individual's concept of self is one of significant loss in regard to body integrity and his total identity. The realization of this loss precipitates reactions of grief and mourning for the previous self, both of which are necessary mechanisms in preventing a complete breakdown of the ego, while adapting to the new disability. Threats to the self-concept become more pronounced when the patient realizes that his sexual identity, as he perceived it, is no longer secure, but seems changed.

It has been found that there is often a wide discrepancy between sexual function of the patient and his sexual identity. For example, one study of spinal cord–injured patients found all levels of remaining functional ability with regard to sex, but all patients experienced some change in sexual identity. This involved changes in their self-esteem with regard to many factors: actual sexual performance, society's imposed roles of masculinity and feminity, and other preconceived ideas about the disabled person's sex roles. Many disabled men feel a humilitating sense of inadequacy (Robmault 1978).

Assessment indicators of sexual dysfunction include the following subjective data:

"I'd be better off dead!"
"What kind of future is there for half a man?"
"What woman would want me?"
"I guess I'll never have a romance again."
"I can't feel anything down 'there'."
"I can't have an erection or ejaculate."

The patient may recite risqué jokes, use profanity, brag about previous sexual experiences, or sexualize the care given by female personnel. Some patients may not verbalize their fears and concerns about their sexual future, but it is safe to assume that they have given the subject considerable thought.

A patient's other reactions to his injury might include acting out behaviors, slamming doors, being demanding of staff, anger (with staff,
family, self), withdrawal or depression, and drying. A multitude of factors
are involved in an individual's reaction to his spinal cord injury. Initially
much energy is utilized in hoping for complete recovery and grieving for
the lost self. Immobility and the ensuing feeling of powerlessness can
devastate the sense of autonomy as well as the sense of manhood (Crigler
1974). The need to disprove these threats to his manhood may be the basis
for the sexual acting-out behavior seen in men with recent injuries,
expressed in jokes, bragging, and profanity. With the return of reflex
activity (if there is return) the patient usually experiences reflex erections.
This occurrence can help bolster a failing male ego. How these events are
managed may well determine whether the patient feels his sexual concerns
are acceptable for discussion or not.

Relationships between the disabled and the significant other (be she wife
or girlfriend) include problems of role changes and role conflict. Many
expectations become incorporated in the gender role performance of certain "valued" tasks. Spinal cord injury interferes with the effective performance of such roles as male breadwinner, sexual partner, and father. The
accepted norm in America for male behavior seems to be aggressive performance in all areas of one's gender role: vocational, recreational, sexual,
and familial. The spinal cord–injured male perceives all these roles to be
terminated; for him the future has little to offer except a complete role
reversal and existence of helpless dependency (Crigler 1974).

Another problem occurs when the disabled individual in effect takes on
the child role and the significant other assumes the parent role. For a quadriplegic man who may need much or all of his personal care done for
him, the significant other becomes the care-giver/parent by feeding,
bathing, and dressing him. It is difficult for some to make the transition
from this role to the one of wife or lover without some problems.

Many couples also find some initial difficulty with the physical role
reversal that may be necessary. Often the female partner must be the dom-
inant partner during the sex act itself. Depending on their previous sexual
activities, this may be psychologically unacceptable. Often both partners
are concerned that their intimacies will cause reinjury. Or, conversely, they
may fear that they are growing apart because the injured partner is so
wrapped up in his needs, losses, and frustrations that he changes from his
accustomed behavior. Also, the healthy partner may be plagued by feelings of guilt that she is able-bodied. She may also harbor anger concerning
the circumstances of the injury or that the disabled individual's injury has
so dramatically changed their lives. Conversely, some women have
expressed a sense of freedom from pressure of sex after their husband's
injury. All of these problems—role reversal, anger, fear, and resentment—

can lead to a decrease in communication and a widening gap between the couple. When there is a decrease in communication and intimacy, decreased sexual activity and satisfaction will ensue.

MANAGEMENT

DIAGNOSTIC PLAN

1. A complete history should be taken and a physical examination made.
2. A neurological examination should be given as described previously (initial and periodically) to assess the level of injury and degree of completeness in order to establish guidelines for intervention.
3. A complete sexual history prior to injury should be taken.
4. A history of sexual activity since injury should be taken.
5. The frequency of erections, duration of erection, if erections are functional for intromission, if ejaculation occurs, and if orgasm is experienced should be ascertained.
6. A sperm count, if obtainable, should be made.

Patient education and counseling are important aspects of treatment of a patient with sexual dysfunction. Some patients benefit from penile prosthetic implants. If a penile prosthetic implant appears appropriate, three implant devices are available. The Small-Carrion device is the most familiar and consists of two sponge-filled silicone rods. The rods have no movable parts and when implanted in the corpora cavernose, they produce sufficient length, width, and girth to simulate the normal erection. One disadvantage is that the penis remains in a state of semi-erection. The second type is very much the same except that it is not as rigid and is on a "hinge" so it is more flexible. This is called the Flexi-Rod. The third device is the inflatable penile prosthesis called the Brantly-Scott. A hollow silicone cylinder is implanted in each corpus cavernosum, a reservoir of radiopaque solution is sutured to the abdominal facsia, and a bulb is implanted in one scrotal sac. The cylinders, reservior and bulb are con nected by silicone tubes. When the patient compresses the bulb in the scrotum, solution flows from the reservior to the cylinder in each corpus cavernosum. The cylinders fill with fluid and an erection occurs. To deflate the cylinder, the patient compresses the release valve in the lower portion of the bulb in the scrotum. The fluid then returns to the reservoir (Wood and Rose 1978).

Surgical complications can occur with penile implants. A thorough history and physical exam must be done, including a complete genitourinary workup. With patients with neurogenic bladders, bladder function must be adequate and the implant must not interfere with its function. Also, the urine should be sterile at the time of surgery to decrease chances of infection. This can be difficult with SCI patients. Patient counseling and education pre- and postoperatively are important. It should be stressed that penile implants make the penis erect but solve no other problems. If the patient was not able to ejaculate prior to the implant, he will still be unable to ejaculate. If he had communication problems with his sex partner, these, too, will still exist. Penile implants may offer a hopeful alternative for some patients, but should not be viewed as a panacea.

The advantages and disadvantages of the types of implants can be summarized as follows:

INFLATABLE TYPE

Advantages

- The erection process simulates normal function, which enhances psychological satisfaction.
- When not erect, the penis assumes normal appearance.
- The length and girth of the penis are greater than with the rod device.
- It does not interfere with urinary function.

Disadvantages

- Surgery is relatively expensive.
- The recovery period is longer than with non-inflatable type.
- Common complications are glans penis inflammation, foreskin tightness, adhesions, kinks or leaks in tubing, reimplantation is sometimes necessary, insertion is complex, and replacement can be difficult.

NON-INFLATABLE TYPE

Advantages

- Surgery is relatively inexpensive.
- Insertion and replacement are relatively simple.
- The recovery period is short.
- There are fewer complications.

Disadvantages

- The penis is constantly semi-erect.
- Concealment is difficult.
- The rod may migrate, fracture, or obstruct the urinary tract.
- The glans penis may slip over prosthesis, requiring reimplantation.
- The dimensions of the penis are smaller than with inflatable type.

Whether or not a patient is a candidate for or chooses to have a penile implant, education and counseling are by far the most important aspects of sexual rehabilitation. Some general guidelines to remember when counselling patients have been outlined by Macrae and Henderson (1975):

Knowledge of normal sexual function and dysfunction is essential.

Knowledge of neurophysiology and the ability to perform and interpret the neurological exam are important.

It is essential for the health professional to come to terms with his/her own sexuality.

The health professional must be aware and in control of his own uncomfortable or unresolved feelings toward patient sexual dysfunction.

No one (patient or health professional) should be forced to discuss sex or related topics that may be anxiety-producing.

Moral, religious and aesthetic considerations need to be respected and accepted.

One's own moral judgments should not enter into counseling of the patient.

All aspects of a relationship, including the sexual, require awareness, communication, and a mutual commitment.

Options should be presented that give the patient and partner freedom to choose what they are most comfortable with.

Know the appropriate resource or referral person should it be necessary.

Often spinal cord–injured patients are given no sex counseling education at all. Part of the problem may be the question of who should counsel. Many times no one person will take the initiative, or the staff will avoid the subject, hoping someone else will take care of it. It is important for the health care team to view sexual rehabilitation as just one part of total rehabilitation of the patient. When this foundation is laid, sexuality can be included with all other health issues and handled in a matter-of-fact manner. Obviously the health care team first needs education and preparation. An active inservice program is a necessity for the entire health care team, as the patient often chooses to confide in the nursing assistant or technician. To keep from overwhelming the patient who is still in the denial stage, the subject of sex should never be presented abruptly. Instead, it should be made clear to the patient that sexuality is an open topic for discussion. The patient is then allowed to initiate the discussion when he is ready. When a patient indicates he is ready to talk about his sexual concerns, he needs some general information. He needs to know how his injury will affect his sexual functioning and what statistics have shown other SCI patients' functioning to be. Emphasis should be on relationships and not on physical acts of intercourse. It must be reinforced that nobody is too disabled to derive some satisfaction from sex. It is important to emphasize that sex is not an all or none experience, and that sexuality has many meanings for different people. If a patient has little or no genital functioning, it does not preclude his experiencing a satisfying, intimate relationship.

There are many ways to counsel patients. These include one-to-one counseling, group sessions, and conjoint sessions. Each patient must be evaluated to determine which method would be most helpful. Some patients aren't able to speak in a group, while others like the support a group gives. It is conceivable that all three methods can be used effectively. One-to-one counseling builds trust, confidence, and assessment of the problem. Group sessions are sometimes good for teaching and support. Conjoint sessions can help the patient to explore a relationship with a significant other.

The key to successful counseling, regardless of the method used, is to establish an atmosphere of concern and acceptance of the patient's feelings. Also, the therapeutic relationship must be based on patience. Allow the patient time to adjust to his condition and feelings. Equally important is confidentiality and privacy. The patient must feel comfortable about discussing his problem and feel that it will be confidential. Counseling should not end after one session, but should be continuous to reinforce success and discuss solutions to new problems. The focus of counseling should always be to increase communication and intimacy between the couple so that they may discover what is mutually satisfying to both. It is almost impossible to separate education and counseling. General education can probably be done well in group sessions. Here, patients are free to ask questions and to respond. It is here that general information can be given about positions, what to do with catheters, bowel difficulty, and other problems that may arise. Specific problems can then be discussed in individual sessions.

Some general information that could be helpful to the patient might include the following:

Sensation.   Much of sexual arousal, excitement, and gratification comes from the stimulation of secondary erogenous zones. Sensation may become acute at the body level just above the sensory loss, and this area may become an area of eroticized skin (Robmault 1978).

Pain.   Any condition that causes pain or discomfort will interfere with sexual response.

Bowel/Bladder.   It is not necessary to remove the catheter from the penis before intercourse; it can be bent over out of the way. Condom catheters can be removed. If the bladder is likely to leak, it can be emptied by crede method before sexual activity. Patients on a regular bowel program are wise to choose a time for sexual activities when their bowels are not expected to move. In all cases common sense is the rule.

Mobility. The individual must face his physiological and anatomical limitations and, while acknowledging what he can no longer do, learn new activities that he can do. The individual with lifelong mobility limitations must also make a realistic assessment of how to function in order to give and receive sexual pleasure (Robmault 1978).

Fantasy. In human beings, fantasy is one of the infinite number of libidinal turn-ons that can be developed for giving and receiving sexual pleasure.

Spasticity. For some patients, spasticity means erective potential. In this case they may need to alter their drug (valium etc.) or ETOH intake prior to intercourse. In some cases spasticity may interfere with sexual function, causing uncontrollable movements that flex or extend the affected parts.

Pressure. No matter what positions are assumed during sexual activity, care must always be taken to prevent pressure sores.

Osteoporosis. Patients with a long-standing injury may develop chronic osteoporosis. Their long bones are easily injured. If the chosen coital position is one in which the patient bears the weight of the partner, the remoral shaft or neck may fracture with relatively little stress. This cannot be reliably predicted or prevented, since the fractures are painless and the precise time of their occurrence often unknown (Horenstein 1976).

Procreation. There have been a few studies in the past 30 years of attempts to obtain semen for analysis and possible artificial insemination. Guttman (1976) cites three methods:

1. Prostatic massage and electrical rectal stimulation
2. Testicular biopsy
3. Intrathecal prostigmin assessment test.

None of these methods is yet reliable or widely used. They present, however, hope for the future.

In summary, sexual function in the male is a complex interaction of spinal cord reflex, supra-spinal influences, and psychological factors. Spinal cord injury can result in impotence. Enervation for sexual function is in the sacral cord levels two, three, and four. Resulting sexual function after injury depends on the level of injury and the completeness of the injury. UMN injuries generally have reflexogenic erections, and incomplete injuries have reflex and some psychogenic erections. LMN complete injuries generally have no erections, and incomplete LMN injuries sometimes have psychogenic erections.

Impotence can greatly alter an already altered body image, adding insult to injury. Spinal cord injury and resultant impotence affect family members and significant others also. Understanding and education are necessary for them as well as for the patient.

Re-education and counseling are very important in the management plan. Surgery for erectile impotence is available to some patients. Gratification for sexual partners can be experienced from feelings other than those emanating from the sex organs during the human sexual response cycle.

At the present time, the probable ability of SCI patients to sire progeny is not too favorable, but alternative methods are being studied. Health professionals treating spinal cord–injured patients need to recognize the potentially devastating effects of impotence. In order to respond therapeutically, they must explore with the patient his feelings regarding his sexuality, psychological well-being, appearance, self-concept, body image, and relationships. They can then together decide on interventions most appropriate for that patient.

NEUROPHYSIOLOGY AND PATHOPHYSIOLOGY OF SEXUAL FUNCTION IN THE FEMALE

The normal human sexual response cycle depends on two physiological processes: vasocongestion and myotomia. Cortical influences, peripheral nerves, autonomic pathways, spinal cord pathways, and reflex centers all play a part in sexual functioning. Male and female external sex organs originate from the same parts in embryonic development. The glans penis and clitoris correspond, the shaft of the penis and the area immediately around and above the clitoris correspond, and the scrotum and major lips correspond (Rabin 1980). The sexual response cycle is classified into four stages: excitement, plateau, orgasm, and resolution. During the excitement stage, caused by touch, vision, or imagination, psychic or physical stimuli are transmitted by descending as well as ascending nerves The excitation must be sufficient and continuous to extend all cycles. Stimuli resulting from pressure or tension in the pelvic organs or from touch applied to the external genitalia excite impulses that are mediated by the pelvic and pudendal nerves. These impulses are carried to the sacral cord where response is felt. Sexual stimuli are then transmitted to the brain. Reflexes important in the female orgasm emanate from the sacral area of the cord. The erectile tissue in the female pelvis is controlled by the parasympathetic nerves parting from the sacral plexus to the genitals. This nervous response produces vasocongestion, vaginal lubrication, thickening of the vaginal walls, elevation of the cervix, engorgement of the clitoris, nipple erection, and a sex flush. During the plateau stage, excitement increases and mucus is secreted immediately inside the vagina. There is discoloration of the genitals, quickened breathing, and increased heart rate The orgasmic phase is concentrated in the clitoris, vagina, and uterus and is capable of multiple occurrences. The rectal and urethral sphincters contract. Body muscles in general contract. There is pelvic response and contraction. After the height of the orgasmic experience, there is a resolution stage returning through plateau and excitement to an unstimulated stage.

As has been previously stated, after injury to the spinal cord, there will be no reflex activity at the level of the injury, but, if the reflex arcs remain intact, there may be a return of reflex activity below the level of injury. Thus the female could experience excitement, plateau, and orgasm. If sensation and movement are lost, this experience is not likely to occur unless there is an incomplete injury or sacral sparring. In essence, the response of SCI women is the same as able-bodied females in all respects except for the pelvic response, tension release, and perceived sensation. The normal response is a two-phase motor type. The first consists of contracting of smooth muscle in the fallopian tubes, uterus, and parauretral tubes. Phase two, the concentration contraction of striated muscles of the pelvic floor, perineum, and anal sphincter, is activated by those nerves in the S2, 3, 4 cord segments. The sensory appreciation of these muscle responses is the basis, in part, for the perception of orgasm. In SCI women, orgasm is rare. There does seem to be a heightened arousal, or paraorgasm, by means of tactile stimulation of an area above the lesion and redesigning that sensation to the genitals. Tactile feeling of these areas is sometimes very intense, particularly around the breast. This supersensitivity is known as hyperesthesia and might contribute to Masters and Johnson's report of breast-oriented orgasm. In these cases, orgasm seems to be highly linked to vivid fantasies or dreams as well as physiological excitations and release (Miller 1979).

Much of the literature suggests a passive sexual role for women and more specifically for the SCI woman. For some women this may be the case, either as a choice to save energy, moral considerations, or societal assimilation. It has been found, however, that oral and manual sex is widely practiced by a great number of SCI females (Rabin 1980). This method seems to afford more active engagement for the more physically restricted female to explore her partner and in turn receive pleasure from her partner in quite specific and direct ways. Positioning in sexual activity is limited only by the amount of energy each partner is willing to exert and by the remaining trunk muscles used for balance. Water or air flotation mattresses contribute to a woman's movement and pleasure. Although menstruation is interrupted about 50 percent of the time, it usually returns within six months. Due to the change in sensation, cramping is usually greatly diminished or absent all together. The SCI woman is just as susceptible to pregnancy as the able-bodied woman. Complications due to urinary tract infections, autonomic dysreflexia, anemia, and premature delivery are possibilities that must be closely monitored. Vaginal delivery is generally allowed when the injury is below the T6 level. Caesarean delivery is usually recommended for higher injuries because of the danger

of autonomic dysreflexia. Uterine involution and milk production following delivery are normal. Episiotomy is acceptable, but daily self-skin
inspections are recommended, and stitching is preferable to stapling.
Women with injuries at the level of T8 and below will experience delivery
pains.

Most women of childbearing age need assistance with family planning.
Two forms of birth control that are contraindicated in the SCI person are
the intrauterine device (IUD) and the pill. IUDs have been known to
migrate in location and to cause severe abdominal cramping. Because of
change in sensation, this warning sign is absent and could cause bodily
injury. The pill is contraindicated in view of the decreased venous circulation and the susceptibility to thrombophlebitis. The use of the condom
with spermicidal jelly is the most effective means of birth control and the
safest, but it may be unacceptable to one or both of those involved.
Women with lesions at or above T-11 will have reflexive activity of the
vaginal secretory glands. Those with injuries below T-11 can be advised to
use some water-soluable lubricant for vaginal lubrication.

PSYCHOSOCIAL CONSIDERATIONS

In considering the topic of sexuality with spinal cord injury (SCI), a dis-
tinction should be made between sex as a physiological capacity for intercourse, and sexuality that goes far beyond the biological factors. Sexuality
involves a female—woman, wife, or mother—and each of these roles
demands that she behave in a particular manner. How she behaves is indicative of how she values herself. Sexuality includes the whole spectrum of
attitudes and is reflected in all parts of a woman, her relationships, and her
activities. People are sexual beings, and this is as true for disabled women
as it is for able-bodied women. Sexuality is one of life's major forces,
which guides and shapes a person's psychological rehabilitation.

Sexual adjustment following SCI is a many-faceted process. The most
prevalent psychological reaction, as with other traumatic injuries, is a reactive depression (Rigoni 1978). It usually proceeds through four basic
stages: shock, denial, acknowledgment, and then adjustment. The stage of
shock allows for very little personal involvement in the corrective sense,
both physically and psychologically. In the denial stage, the woman
believes her injury is only temporary and she will be as she was before.
Anger sometimes vents itself toward the end of this stage as a defense
against the constant confrontations of reality. She may also be very upset
with her physical condition and the many questions she is beginning to
formulate regarding her social self, and therefore she projects this anger
outwardly. While this action usually alienates many of her care-givers, it is
considered to be a positive step, as it indicates the beginning of acknowledgment and the road to maximum recovery.

The stage of acknowledgment may be accompanied by increased depth of depression as the woman who desires independence begins to realize her need for help or dependency. Sexual fears surface at this stage. She begins to wonder about her self-worth, attractiveness, and sexual potential. In general, she may find herself having to define herself as a woman. She has to adjust to a new self-image. As her functional abilities increase, so will her self-worth. Many women do not progress to this stage of adjustment for many months, and some may take years to work through the experience. If the situation seems too difficult and her resources are too few, the woman may turn to drugs of one type of another to displace the anxiety. Suicide is a major killer of SCI persons during this stage. The striving for physical and psychological independence can result in frustration, hostility, and even withdrawal. The balance between acceptance of dependence and attaining a degree of independence is a critical point in her psychological adjustment and the building up of self-esteem. Patients with premorbid personalities make poor adjustments. This, however, does not mean that a woman who has experienced confusion or uncertainty in this area can never adjust.

When the woman is able to recognize that she has many things to offer the world, her family, her friends and, more important, her lover, her increased self-esteem helps her cope with her inadequacies. Common concerns of women regardless of injuries include attractiveness, employment, fertility, mothering ability, harmony in her environment, sexual potential, and being happy and fulfilled. Not being able to feel that she has something to offer in these areas results in diminished self-worth and affects the rehabilitation of a woman with SCI (Cole 1979).

Sexuality encompasses the entire spectrum of relating to another person: the smiles, the friendships, the touches, the giving, the receiving, and the tolerances and frustrations as well. Assertiveness, confidence, and communication are essential ingredients of a more complete identity. The need to say what one likes or doesn't like with regard to others' feelings is an essential part of expressing sexuality. The therapist should not push his or her attitudes and desires on the patient. Rehabilitation is promoted by a relationship that is based on respect and consideration for the individuality and feelings of the injured person. This climate is also most conducive to the patient feeling free to ask questions and to discuss her concerns.

10

Vascular Disorders

MARGARET FORD and MARGARET ANN SEVERSON

Vascular disease encompasses several disordered states and is not to be taken lightly. Terms used to identify it include deep vein thrombosis (DVT), thrombophlebitis, phlebothrombosis, and pulmonary embolism (PE).

Thrombophlebitis is defined as an occlusion of a vein in which the inflammatory process occurs first and the thrombosis second. Phlebothrombosis occurs when the thrombosis is primary and inflammation secondary (Ryan 1978). Clinically, it is extremely difficult to differentiate between the two. Therefore, in this chapter the two terms, along with the term DVT, will be used interchangeably. Pulmonary embolism (thromboembolism) is defined as the lodgement of a blood clot in a pulmonary artery with subsequent obstruction of blood supply to the lung parenchyma. The course of the disease is always an ominous one, but it is particularly so in the spinal cord–injured patient. The absence or decrease of skin sensation, immobilization, and flaccid extremities, among other factors, renders this type of patient a prime target for venous disease. Another important factor that predisposes to venous disease is the fact that subjective symptoms so vital in early diagnosis cannot be experienced by the patient with paralysis.

INCIDENCE, EPIDEMIOLOGY, ETIOLOGY, AND PATHOPHYSIOLOGY

The incidence of DVT in the SCI population varies from 12 percent by clinical and radiological diagnosis, to 61 percent using impedance plethysmography and contrast venography, to 100 percent by I. Fibrinogen uptake. Pulmonary embolism from thrombophlebitis occurs in 5 to 10 percent of the SCI population with a mortality rate of 2 to 10 percent, with some studies showing a mortality as high as 20 percent (Falotico 1979).

With new diagnostic techniques, it has been shown that one out of every three patients develops thrombosis in calf veins within 36 hours after major surgery or trauma. Clinically, only one out of seven cases is apparent. Fibrin deposits are detectable in 50 percent of SCI by the end of the second post-injury week and in all patients by the fourth week (Maurice 1974).

Studies have shown that a higher incidence of complications from thrombophlebitis occurs with a complete spinal cord lesion as opposed to incomplete lesions. Dorsal lesions in particular are higher in incidence than cervical or thoracic levels. However, in terms of death due to complication of thrombophlebitis, cervical injuries are at highest risk [Perkash et al. 1979; Watson 1978].

As to the site of the disease, it is estimated that at least 70 percent of all cases of thrombophlebitis occurred in the left leg, 10 percent in the pelvic veins, and the remaining 20 percent were unidentifiable in terms of localization. They were, however, definitely not localized in the right leg as indicated by absent signs and symptoms in the right leg (Hachen 1974). The reason for the absence of right leg involvement in not known. Research carried out in England demonstrated that approximately 90 percent of the complications of deep vein thrombosis in spinal cord injury occurred within a month after injury. Specifically, the second and third weeks within that first month were the most common time of onset (Watson 1978). Factors such as age, weight, and/or surgical procedures had no significant bearing on the development of venous disease in this study. Other studies have implicated age over 50, obesity, and surgical procedures as contributing to venous disease.

The majority of the occurrences of calf vein thrombosis are asymptomatic. If untreated, however, 20 percent will extend into proximal veins, which include popliteal, femoral, and iliac veins. Fifty percent of these will embolize to the lungs (Turpie and Hirsh 1980).

It is assumed that the etiology of thrombus formation in a spinally injured person is similar to that occurring in any patient. This assumption includes the presence of a sluggish venous circulation and lower extremities being in a flaccid state. Additional factors that contribute to the risk for a SCI patient are (a) hypercoagulable state, (b) long duration of immobility, and (c) an abnormality of the vein wall. The patient with a cord injury, by the very nature of his trauma, is in a hypercoagulable state that is considerably greater than that of the normal post-surgical patient (Perkash et al. 1979; Watson 1978). The almost constant presence of urinary tract infections of spinal cord–injured patients triggers intravascular clotting due to the presence of endotoxins in the blood. Gram-negative bacteria have a thrombogenic effect and enter the venous circulation from the urinary bladder (Weiss 1977). Deep pelvic veins are especially vulnerable to thrombogenic effects of gram-negative bacteria in urinary tract infections entering the venous circulation via the bladder (Perkash et al. 1979). This state of hypercoagulation in the SCI patient peaks at the end of the first month after injury and again at the end of the third month (Dollin 1980).

The long duration of immobility in bed results in up to 50 percent reduction in blood flow to the extremities and increased vasodilation and venous pooling. The risk is enhanced by pressure of the calf muscles against the bed. Other conditions that increase the risk are congestive heart failure, compression of the veins by tumor, distension of the abdomen, and the flaccid state of paralyzed limbs from failure of an active calf pump. The absence of the active calf muscle pump, normally present in the healthy extremity, increases the incidence of impaired venous return and stasis that results from the calf resting against the bed. The muscle tone in the lower extremities also appears to play a role in the development of venous disease, with increasing vulnerability at the time of return in spasticity.

Damage to the endothelium of the vein causes an interruption in its usual smooth surface. Platelets and other debri adhere to the resulting rough surface, and the clotting process begins. This occurs with varicose veins, previous DVT, and with trauma to the vein wall. Intravenous injections, surgery, and complicated deliveries are the most common causes of trauma.

A thrombus is an inflammation of the lining of the vein with clot formation at the site of tissue injury. Thrombi are usually classed according to anatomic location, as superficial, deep, or a combination of these. In superficial thrombi, the greater saphenous vein is the most common site, usually at the sinus of the valves. Along the length of the involved vein there is considerable pain, tenderness, and redness. Swelling is evident as the disease progresses and the vein becomes firm and hard. There is no generalized edema because the deep venous system continues to function. This reduces venous engorgement and fluid transudation from the capillary bed into extravascular tissues (Krupp and Chattam 1978; Price and Wilson 1978).

In deep thrombophlebitis, generalized edema is caused by obstructed venous flow. The following three areas are most likely to become involved: the iliofemoral vein, the femoropopliteal segment, and the small veins of the calves. When the calf veins alone are involved, there is usually no propagation of the thrombus beyond the margin of the valve cusps. As one might expect, symptoms vary greatly depending on location and the extent of the thrombus and the extent of the occlusion. One of the most ominous developments mentioned earlier is the incidence of pulmonary emboli. These are the thrombi that detach themselves from the vein wall, enter the circulation, and lodge in the lung tissue, a situation to be avoided at all costs. One important thing for the health practitioner to bear in mind is that all the above-mentioned signs may not be present in deep vein thrombosis. Edema, increased calf girth, and local deep tenderness are the most reliable physical signs, but even these cannot be relied upon (Krupp and Chattam 1978).

The main cellular components in a thrombus are platelets, leucocytes, and red blood cells. These are held together by fibrin, a protein formed in complex stages from the plasma protein, fibrinogen. Thrombi are classified structurally as simple or mixed. The composition of simple thrombus is basically one element—either platelet, fibrin, or red cell. *Platelet thrombi* are usually found in small vessels, arterioles, and cardiac valves. The platelets are closely packed, forming aggregates. They do not, as a rule, develop into larger, more complex lesions, as there is no opportunity for growth. So there is little likelihood of the development of a large embolus. The other type of thrombi, however, are especially known for their progression into lethal emboli (Price and Wilson 1978).

Fibrin thrombi are distinctly different from the other types. Composed of mostly fibrin strands, they are closely packed and occur almost exclusively in the capillary beds. There are a few platelets in these masses, and they may or may not be aggregated. Their arrangement is such that they appear to be trapped in the fibrin strands.

The third type of simple thrombus is the *red cell type*. They have been observed, in vivo, in arterioles, venules, and capillaries. They are usually agglutinated. Sickle cell anemia is a prime example of red cell aggregation.

Mixed thrombi form in arteries, veins, and heart tissue. They may be of any size and usually include all the main elements: platelets, leucocytes, and fibrin. A recognizable pattern forms the structural unit. The aggregated platelets, membranes intact, are surrounded by fibrin and leucocytes. Red blood cells make up the bulk of the thrombus, and fibrin strands connect one unit to another unit.

All of these thrombi are formed in one of two ways: on an injured vessel wall as a mural thrombus, or in the bloodstream. It is theorized that the thrombi formed in the bloodstream separate from the stream and attach to endothelial tissue at the site of injury. Platelets are the first to separate from the flowing blood and bind at the damaged-tissue site. More platelets adhere to these and an aggregate is formed. One can conclude that disturbances in the rate of blood flow can account for one type of clot formation, and tissue injury accounts for the other type. It is easy to see why the spinal cord–injured patient is susceptible to both (Perkash et al. 1979; Van Hove 1978; Watson 1978).

MAJOR PSYCHOSOCIAL COMPONENTS AND FAMILIAL
IMPACT OF THE DIAGNOSIS

Spinal cord injury presents a long and arduous struggle for the continuation of a meaningful life. This is true not only for the person who has sustained the injury, but also for family and significant others. Anything that prolongs this struggle means further devastation to the already burdened people involved. When the long period of immobilization is increased for any reason, the patient is jeopardized physically and emotionally. A successful adjustment to the injury can be significantly or even permanently delayed (Weiss 1977).

It is generally agreed that the manner in which we experience any disability depends primarily on four factors: (a) physical factors, (b) psychological factors, (c) circumstances not related to the disability, and (d) the comparison with able-bodied people. This belief is further expanded to include the stages of illness experienced by the paralyzed person: (a) shock, (b) anger, (c) disbelief, (d) depression, and (e) adjustment. These stages parallel those theorized in the Kübler-Ross approach to the person dealing with loss. Yet some aspects of these stages are peculiar to the person with a profound trauma and major change in body image. The impact of thrombophlebitis on the beleaguered patient is greatly determined by the pre-morbid personality and the state of adaptation to the SCI at the time of onset. Studies show that the last stage of adaptation—adjustment— is the one in which a setback is least tolerated, because this is usually when the patient begins life in a wheelchair. In other words, he has just begun "ambulation," and to be reconfined to bed for venous disease or any other problem at this stage can produce pathological reactions (Weiss 1977).

With the presence of DVT or PE, the rehabilitation and adjustment process is delayed. Further immobility and dependency are placed on the patient in the acute phase of his venous disease, often leading to depression and boredom. The patient and his family are already dealing with the initial spinal cord injury and often become overwhelmed by the threat of PE. PE brings fear because of its fatal implications as well as fear of its treatment, which could cause severe hemorrhage. The patient's and family's response to the development of venous disease will greatly depend on their stage of adjustment in regard to the primary illness. Successful rehabilitation of the spinal cord–injured individual ultimately depends on psychosocial adaptations. Although patients are ultimately responsible for their own adjustment, they are often adversely affected by those around them. Support from family and significant others plays an important role in the SCI patient's motivation for recovery and return to the community. It is essential that those around him adopt healthy role expectations for the patient and help him to fulfill them.

SUBJECTIVE AND OBJECTIVE PHYSICAL DATA

A systematic, organized approach is important in gathering subjective and objective data leading to the diagnosis of venous disease. Subjective symptoms are rarely heard from the spinal cord–injured patient with phlebitis. The devious nature of clot formation, plus the lack of sensation in the lower extremities, makes the presence of venous disease difficult if not impossible for the patient to detect.

The physical examination begins with inspection of the lower extremities. The patient should be exposed foot to groin. The practitioner observes for asymmetric enlargement, especially in the calf regions. Calf and thigh measurements should be done daily and recorded. Differences of 15 mm in men and 12 mm in women are diagnostic of thrombophlebitis 80 percent of the time (Ryan 1978). With DVT, the superficial veins are usually distended because they carry much of the venous return when the deep veins are obstructed. They can best be seen in the dorsal foot veins, anterior tibial, or knee regions. Unless the extremity is elevated 45 degrees, dilated dorsal foot veins are not significant as a positive indication of DVT. Anterior tibial vein dilation is significant and may be observed only in the dependent position (Ryan 1978). Also observe the color of the extremity, noting erythemia. Cyanosis may be seen in the lower third of the leg if DVT is present.

Prior to palpation, practitioner should place his hands in cool water for a few minutes to increase the perceptiveness of the hands to the temperature rise that occurs with thrombosis. Change in temperature of the affected extremity may be one of the first objective signs of DVT. The interval between the appearance of warmth and the development of other signs of DVT varies from one to seven days, the average being three days. Deep palpation is the most discriminating test. The patient's legs are flexed at the knee and the examination initiated at the achilles tendon, proceeding to the popliteal region. If a DVT is present, a tender cordline thrombosis segment will be palpable. Then the practitioner palpates the lower medial thigh extending to the femoral region in the groin. The exact location and progression of the thrombosed vein can be monitored daily.

During the physical exam, some clinicians use a maneuver to aid in clot detection. Tourniquets are applied at successive points along the leg to aid in observation of variations in the timing and direction of filling of the superficial veins during dependency. This is done immediately following elevation of the extremity. It permits detection and localization of incompetent valves (Price and Wilson 1978). If pain sensation can be felt, the examiner can differentiate venous tenderness from muscle tenderness. Venous involvement is noted when fingertip palpation causes greater pain that lateral compression of the calf (Hume 1976).

Although not always applicable to the spinal cord injured, other clinical examination signs can be used in early diagnosis of DVT. They refer to tenderness and pain in the lower extremities. Generally, the greater the degree of local tenderness, the less is the danger of embolism because thrombi usually loosen before a pronounced inflammatory process develops. The following tests would be used primarily in the patient with an incomplete lesion who has sensation in his lower extremities:

Homan's sign is one of the best known and commonly used signs in detecting DVT. It is done by a forceful abrupt dorsiflexion of the foot while the knee is flexed. A positive sign occurs only when pain is elicited in both popliteal and calf regions. In one study, a positive Homan's sign was diagnostically helpful in less than 50 percent of the cases. Other conditions may cause a false positive result (Ryan 1978).

Ranirez's sign is one of the most significant signs of the presence of DVT. With the patient in a recumbent position with the leg flexed, a sphygmomanometer cuff is placed above the knee with a pressure of 40 mmHg. The venous hypertension produced will cause pain in the popliteal or calf regions in the presence of DVT. The pain will disappear instantaneously as the cuff is released. It is important to release the cuff slowly because rapid release in the presence of venous hypertension may cause thrombi to dislodge from the vessel wall, leading to PE and death (Ryan 1978).

Bancroft's sign is done by compression of the calf in an anterior posterior direction or against the tibia. A positive pain response indicates deep phlebitis only when the pain is greater than that experienced from Moser's sign. *Moser's sign* is looked for in lateral compression with the gastrocnemius lifted away from the tibia. Greater tenderness on lateral compression than anterior posterior compression indicates involvement of the muscle rather than the veins (Ryan 1978).

Lowenberg's sign is elicited with blood pressure cuffs wrapped around both calves. With inflation, the pressure is noted at which pain in each leg is experienced. Normally the patient will not feel discomfort below 180 mmHg, but with phlebitis he will usually complain of pain between 60 and 150 mmHg.

Popkin's sign is elicited by pressure of the index finger or thumb over the anterior medial aspect of the lower extremity. This test is a diagnostic aid in detecting stasis from obstruction or venous insufficiency. A positive sign is manifested by a complaint of pain or facial grimaces (Ryan 1978).

Louvel's sign is pain in the leg after coughing or sneezing. The pain is caused by an increase in venous pressure from the cough or sneeze, which is transmitted to the leg veins at the site of the clot.

Pulmonary embolus is also difficult to diagnose in the high level SCI. The

SCI masks the symptoms of chest pain, cough, or hemolysis. In the non-SCI patient, a DVT may be a clue to future PE, but 50 percent of the reported PE in SCI patients had silent DVT. Initially there is a low PO2 accompanying PE, but even in the absence of PE, the SCI has a low PO2 secondary to respiratory muscle paralysis. In general, a PO2 of 80 mmHg or less is accepted for diagnosis of PE; however, an acute quadriplegic may have a PO2 of 70 mmHg or less before the onset of PE, which renders the criteria ineffective for diagnostic purposes. Often severe neck and chest injuries prohibit a perfusion lung scan. A chest X-ray, serial dilution protamine sulfate test, and LDH estimation are helpful in diagnosing such patients (Perkash et al. 1979).

The paraplegic patient will feel the pain that may accompany PE. There may be a sudden onset of dyspnea with a deep, crushing, shooting, knife-like pain that covers the sixth dermatome band reaching, maximal intensity beneath the sternum and aggravated by respiratory motions (Clark 1975). The pain that accompanies a PE is either from the embolus lodging in the pulmonary branches that causes pain in the vessel wall, a decreased cardiac output with decreased blood flow through the coronary arteries causing myocardial pain, or from a decreased blood supply to the pleural tissues. The patient will feel no relief with rest, but the pain is eased with narcotics.

Other symptoms of PE include anxiety, disorientation, hypotension, cyanosis, fever, hemoptysis, weakness, sweating, rales, tachypnea, nausea and vomiting, venous distension in the neck, sinus tachycardia or an irregular cardiac rhythm, narrowly split S2 with accentuation of P2, a gallop or systolic murmur, or a left parasternal heave. The effects of PE depend on the size of the occluded pulmonary artery. The circulation beyond the site of the obstruction is blocked and leads to a reduced blood flow through the lungs to enter the left heart and systemic circulation. Blood dams up behind the area of obstruction and results in necrosis in the area supplied by the occluded pulmonary artery. PE leads to pulmonary hypertension, which leads to acute cor-pulmonale (cor-pulmonale means heart disease secondary to lung disease), reduced cardiac output, hypotension and shock (Young 1976).

To summarize the physical examination, the practitioner is looking for any obvious swelling, local hyperthermia, pain or tenderness. Calf and thigh circumference measurements are done daily at a fixed time until the patient is out of the acute phase of his injury. As a general rule, any change in circumference greater than 1.5 cm needs further evaluation. If the patient is showing clinical signs of PE, arterial blood gases, chest X-ray and lung scan, if not contraindicated, should be done, as described below.

MANAGEMENT PLAN

DIAGNOSTIC TOOLS

All patients need the following tests to determine the presence or the absence of venous disease:

1. A complete blood count, including differential and platelet count
2. A coagulation profile, including an APTT (activated partial thrombo-plastin time), a PT (prothrombin time), and a thrombin time. Normal range for APTT is 25 to 40 seconds, and 11 to 14 seconds for the PT (Daly 1972).
3. Chest X-ray
4. An initial electrical impedance plethysmography, and at weekly intervals while confined to bed
5. Laboratory enzyme studies to determine elevation of LDH and SGOT
6. For some patients, blood gases to detect low pO2.

Diagnostic tools to determine the presence of thrombophlebitis include iodine-labeled fibrinogen leg scan, also known as Fibrinogen Uptake Test (FUT), Dippler Ultrasound Flow Detection (UFD), Impedance Plethys-mography (IPG), and venography (also called phlebography). In diagnos-ing PE, a lung scan, arterial blood gases, and pulmonary angiography are necessary. Each of these tools will be briefly discussed:

1. *Fibrogen Uptake Test,* accurate in early detection of venous obstruc-tion in the calf as opposed to thrombi already formed. This test detects the active thrombosis by measuring and locating the isotope incorporated in the clot. Recordings are made daily for one week, thus day-to-day changes in the size of the thrombus are provided. Thrombus is suspected if there is an increase in radioactivity of 20 percent or more. Since results may not become positive for 72 hours, this test is ineffective in emergency situations.
2. *Doppler Ultrasound,* a noninvasive technique that can be done at the bedside to detect changes in velocity of the venous blood flow. This test screens for femoral thrombosis, and the results may be read in two or three minutes. It is not 100 percent accurate, since venous obliteration must be 50 percent to indicate thrombosis.
3. *Impedance Plethysmography* is a noninvasive test to measure the speed of peripheral drainage after previous venous occlusion. This test is highly sensitive to larger proximal thrombos (i.e., popliteal, femoral, iliac) but insensitive to calf thrombosis. This is a time-consuming test and is often replaced by the Doppler Ultrasound.

4. *Venography* is the most accurate method of diagnosing thrombosis and its location. A radiopaque contrast medium is injected into a vein in the foot to specify the deep venous system of the leg. Abnormalities are seen as contrast filling defects, abrupt termination of a column of contrast, non-filling of a deep venous system despite adequate venographic technique, and the presence of collateral veins. Venography should be done in all cases requiring enzymatic thrombolysis or thrombectomy. The disadvantage of this test is that it is suitable only in deep vein screening. Complications include pain in the legs during injection and, rarely, a hypersensitivity reaction. The occurrence of DVT following venography is rare (Turpie and Hirsh 1980).

Although a negative lung scan almost always rules out PE, pulmonary angiography is the definite diagnostic procedure for confirming PE. It must be done within 36 hours of the onset of clinical symptoms, otherwise a false negative may show resulting from clot lysis.

PREVENTION AND PROPHYLAXIS

In prevention, the three mechanisms responsible for initiating thrombophlebitis must be reduced or eliminated.

1. Measures to avoid venous stasis and/or increase the velocity of blood flow include:

   a. Exercise by rhythmical stimulation of the blood vessels in the calves. Press the patient's feet in a walking action against a foot board in bed and do passive range of motion for ten minutes every two hours.

   b. If a trapeze is used, be sure the patient is taught the correct usage: to exhale during its use. Improper use occurs when the patient closes his glottis and raises his intrathoracic pressure as he pulls himself up in bed. This stimulates the vagus nerve and precipitates arrhythmias. Blood from the inferior vena cava is prevented from emptying into the right atrium, resulting in increased venous pressure and stasis of blood in the lower extremities.

   c. When the patient is sitting on the edge of the bed, feet should be resting firmly on the floor. The legs must not dangle, because the mattress edge pressing against the popliteal space shuts off the venous flow.

   d. If the patient sits for long periods, encourage flexion of the calf muscles to promote venous return. Elevate the legs ten minutes every two hours.

e. Use elastic stockings or ace bandages to suppress flow in the superficial veins and to force blood into the deeper veins to increase the rate of venous blood flow. Also useful is intermittent calf compression and electrical calf muscle stimulation.

f. Encourage deep breathing to promote venous return by a pumping effect exerted on the veins by changes in thoracic pressure.

g. Place a pillow between the legs when side-lying to prevent circulatory pooling of blood from pressure of the bony prominences against the soft tissues.

h. If the feet are elevated, place support along the entire length of the leg. This is best accomplished by raising the foot of the bed eight inches on blocks.

i. Keep the knees higher than the hips to promote venous return.

j. The patient must never sit in a jackknife position, as this causes stasis of blood in the pelvic region.

Patient teaching to reduce venous stasis includes:

- weight reduction
- stopping smoking. The nicotine reduces the caliber of the veins, predisposing them to clot formation
- avoiding restrictive devices around the legs, such as garters, girdles and knee-high stockings
- discouraging patient from crossing his knee.

2. Measures to avoid endothelial injury to the vessels include:

a. Care in intravenous administration. One of the most common sites of injury is the needle insertion site for intravenous treatment. Since many intravenous drugs irritate the vessels secondary to their concentration, and because of the patient's length of exposure to the drug, proper dilution is necessary.

b. Stabilize the indwelling catheter to avoid intravascular trauma. Change the intravenous site every 72 hours. Heparin locks can be changed every fourth day.

c. If the patient is convulsing, restless, or combative, pad the side rails to prevent vessel damage.

3. Measures to reduce or eliminate hypercoagulability include:

a. Be aware of patients prone to thrombosis.

b. Know normal lab values for coagulation times, red and white blood count, sedimentation rate, and values anticipated with optimal anticoagulant therapy.

c. The aim of prophylaxis and treatment of thrombosis is to lower the coagulability of the blood and thus prevent its occurrence, recurrence, propagation and/or embolism of the thrombus.

An unsettled point remains as to the choice of anticoagulant and the period prophylaxis should be maintained. Should anticoagulants cover only the high-risk period of four weeks post-injury, or twelve weeks following injury (this being the period when the majority of patients develop thromboemboli), or simply until wheelchair activity is resumed? Although the majority of acute SCI patients develop DVT within twelve weeks of injury, some continue to be susceptible. Three percent develop DVT after oral anticoagulants are discontinued at twelve weeks. At present, there is no modality to screen out the patients with extended hypercoagulability, and a fixed regime of arbitrary period of prophylaxis may not cover the risk factors in all patients. Therapy, therefore, has to be individualized. Some practitioners do not believe the mortality rate is high enough to justify the routine use of prophylactic anticoagulants.

TREATMENT

The duration of treatment following a DVT is a minimum of ten days, as this is the time required for thrombi to be covered by endothelium and be rendered inactive for propagation. The main objective is to prevent thromboembolism, which is affected primarily by factors of coagulation and is therefore susceptible to modification by anticoagulants. This is opposed to arterial thrombus, in which platelet aggregation factors have more effect, and which is therefore more susceptible to modification by platelet aggregation inhibitors (Rocha et al. 1976). Platelet aggregates at the site of origin of venous thrombus suggest platelets do play a role in initiation of this process. Drugs that suppress platelet function may be of value in the prevention of some high-risk patients (Turpie and Hirsh 1980). Platelet-suppressant drugs include aspirin, dipyridamole, sulfinpyrazone, and hydroxychloroquine. Intravenous heparin is administered initially. It has been shown to prevent factor X activation, a major factor in the coagulation mechanism. It normalizes platelet adhesiveness and inhibits intrinsic thromboplastin generation. Some studies show a 10-day course for the severely injured is insufficient to assure adequate antithrombotic protection and that three weeks is often necessary. In DVT, the range of heparin administration is between 25,000 to 45,000 units per 24 hours. For PE, the initial treatment is with higher doses: 60,000 to 120,000 units per 24 hours, followed by a reduction to 20,000 to 45,000 units per 24 hours (Perkash 1980). The protocol is flexible, but generally it is recommended that the treatment begin with a 2,000 to 5,000 unit bolus, followed by a constant infusion rate of 14 units per kg of body weight per hour (about 1,000 units per hour or 24,000 units in 24 hours). An APTT is done before starting treatment and again two or three hours after initiation of treatment and after each change in heparin dosage. Therefore, it is repeated once daily.

During the last three to five days, heparin therapy is overlapped with the oral anticoagulant Coumadin. Coumadin acts in the liver, interfering with the vitamin K dependent synthesis of factors II, VII, IX, and X. Heparin is discontinued after effective anticoagulation with Coumadin, which occurs with a PT twice the control value. PT is done daily for the first week until the Coumadin dose is stabilized, and weekly or biweekly thereafter. Twelve weeks are recommended for Coumadin therapy following an uncomplicated or moderate DVT, and six months to one year for an extensive DVT or PE. Recurring PE may require even more prolonged treatment of one to two years.

Fibrinolytic therapy with streptokinase and urokinase is utilized for treatment of "massive" PE and DVT. Resolution of emboli is accelerated, but there may be no change in the mortality rate (Freitag and Miller 1980). Bleeding complications are more frequent, more severe, and more difficult to reverse than with heparin treatment. In the presence of PE, oxygen by nasal cannula or face mask may be given in a concentration that maintains the PO2 at or above 60 mmHg. Respirator therapy may be required. Blood pressure and cardiac output must be supported as necessary.

In up to 20 percent of patients with PE, inferior vena cava interruptions with intracaval devices have been required (Freitag and Miller 1980). Indications for this include (a) a precarious clinical state, i.e., massive PE such that another emboli would likely be lethal, (b) high risk for complications with anticoagulants, e.g., bleeding ulcers, reembolization, and (c) septic emboli. Methods of interruption include ligation, plication, placement of an umbrella filter, or clipping of the inferior vena cava. Intracaval devices filter the flood flow, trapping and preventing emboli from traveling to and lodging in the pulmonary arterial tree. The device is placed below the renal portion of the inferior vena cava (Coon 1974). Embolectomy is done only in patients who are hypotensive secondary to an emboli and when it can be accomplished within several hours of the embolic event (Coon 1974).

In the first 72 hours following diagnosis of a DVT or PE, range of motion is withheld. After 72 hours, gentle range of motion of all joints is allowed to prevent contractures. Activity gradually increases after the first week when adequate anticoagulation is established and there is no evidence of progressive active thrombosis (Perkash et al. 1979).

COMPLICATIONS OF ANTICOAGULANT THERAPY

In the use of anticoagulant treatment the practitioner must remember that any substance capable of preventing thrombus formation may lead to severe hemorrhagic complications. Another point to consider is that in the event of severe hemorrhage while on Coumadin treatment, a prescription of vitamin K has no immediate effect. The patient will continue to bleed until plasma levels of the previously depressed clotting factors reach a protective range of 30 to 40 percent (Burke and Murray 1975).

Oral anticoagulants have a narrow range between ineffective, effective, and an overdose. The dosage may be unpredictable from patient to patient and even within the same patient from time to time.

Anticoagulation with Coumadin is dependent on the integrity of the patient's liver function and on vitamin K. Anything that will affect the liver function (e.g., hepatitis) or the level of vitamin K (e.g., alternations in normal bowel flora or decrease or cessation of food intake) will alter the patient's coagulation status. If not corrected, this may lead to fatal hemorrhagic or thrombolic episodes. Anyone involved in administration of Coumadin should be familiar with drug interactions listed in the drug literature.

Drug interactions are rare with heparin, but aspirin should not be given simultaneously. For patients on heparin, their platelets are the only components providing homeostasis, and aspirin inhibits platelet aggregation and prolongs bleeding time. Some practical advantages of heparin administration rather than Coumadin are as follows:

	Heparin	Coumadin
Dosage	Fixed time-dose schedule	Individually adjusted
Therapeutic level	Within 1–2 hours	Within 36–48 hours
Biological half-life	4–5 hours	Close to 24 hours
Laboratory monitoring	Not required	Obligatory
Hemorrhagic complications	Exceptional/ usually benign	Frequent/often severe
Drug compensations	Rapid (protamine)	Slow (Vitamin K)
Drug interactions	Practically unknown	Very common

Some authors regard spinal cord injury as a contraindication to early prophylaxis treatment because of the danger of a small amount of bleeding that may take place in the spinal cord (Silver 1970). The SCI patient on anticoagulation has also been shown to have a higher incidence of ectopic ossification around the hips, possibly owing to bleeding into the adductor muscles. Contraindications to anticoagulant therapy include hemothorax, gastric and duodenal ulcers, severe renal liver disease, uncontrolled hypertension, and head injury. A bleeding episode, per se, is not an indication for discontinuance of anticoagulants. The practitioner and patient must weigh the risk of thromboembolism against the risk of hemorrhage.

PATIENT EDUCATION

Teaching must be individualized for each patient, taking into consideration certain principles of learning, which include:

1. A learner must be physically ready to learn.
2. A learner must be emotionally motivated to learn and be willing to become involved in the learning process.
3. Teaching must build upon the patient's present field of knowledge, range of experience, and interests.
4. Fatigue decreases concentration span.
5. Meaningful repetition reinforces learning.
6. Anxiety may increase interest, but may lessen retention.
7. People learn best by starting with the familiar and working toward the unfamiliar.
8. Praise increases motivation and achievement, and may assist in the transfer of learning from one area to another.
9. Praise, not reproof, provides greater motivation for achievement.
10. Moving from the simple to the complex promotes better learning and gives the learner a sense of accomplishment.
11. Different people learn more easily through different modalities. Appealing to several senses reinforces learning.
12. The environment can be manipulated to increase or decrease learning.
13. People learn by doing.
14. Learning is a continuous process.
15. Start where the patient is and consider the level of ability to learn.

Implementing these principles is one of the major factors in the success of any teaching program in terms of behavior change.

Some of the things a patient should be taught include a simple explanation of the clotting mechanism, how the anticoagulant treatment interferes with this process, the name and dose of the antigoagulant being taken, the importance of wearing or carrying identification indicating the name and dosage of the anticoagulant, information about routine blood work that is periodically required, symptoms that need reporting to the patient's practitioner, and directions regarding diet and drug restrictions.

11

Para-Articular Ossification

JANE EGAN and JEANNE STACK

Para-articular ossification (PAO) was first mentioned by Riedel in 1883 and first studied by Dejerine and her co-workers in 1918 and 1919. Various articles in the literature have dealt with the appearance of soft ossification and have attempted to describe and delineate the problem. The various studies of the disorder have led to the use of several terms. These are myositis ossificans, heterotrophic ossification, dystrophic ossification, paraosteoarthropathy, and para-articular ossification. Since the disorder involves the formation of bone in soft tissue next to normally placed bone, it seems most appropriate to use the term para-articular ossification (Freehafer 1966; Guttmann 1976).

EPIDEMIOLOGY AND PATHOPHYSIOLOGY

The literature indicates the incidence of para-articular ossification is not strictly confined to traumatic paraplegia, although it is most commonly seen in this population. Other neurological disorders that have gross disturbances of spinal cord reflex activity may also have accompanying para-articular ossification. This chapter will focus only on para-articular ossification in relation to the spinal cord–injured person.

Para-articular ossification has been observed in both complete and incomplete paraplegics and quadriplegics in soft tissue. Its occurrence is not related to the spasticity or to the severity of the lesion. Characteristic sites for formation are the hips, shoulders, and elbows. The age of onset can vary from 15 years to 68 years, with the majority occurring from 20 years to 45 years (Hernandez et al. 1978; Scher 1976). Patients under 35 years of age who develop PAO within six months of their injury have a greater incidence of ankylosis (Wharton and Morgan 1970)

Statistics report that between 16 and 49 percent of the spinal cord–injured population form para-articular ossification. Some authorities in the field believe that when all parameters are investigated and documentation is carefully done, the truer incidence is between 20 to 25 percent (Wharton and Morgan 1975). The earliest documented case of para-articular ossification appeared 19 days after injury. However, "the time of peak incidence is during the first six months post trauma . . . lesions may appear as late as twelve to eighteen months post trauma" (Freehafer 1966).

Clinically, four stages of para-articular ossification are evident. Negative radiographic results accompanied by swelling and an elevated serum alkaline phosphatase level characterize stage one. In stage two, positive radiographic findings will be apparent. Serum alkaline phosphatase levels remain elevated with continued swelling. Characteristically, serum alkaline phosphatase begins to come down in stage three but still remains slightly elevated. Findings from radiographic studies reveal positive results. Finally, in stage four, serum alkaline phosphatase levels return to normal; radiographic findings remain positive.

The exact etiology is unknown. Various theories include the following: overly enthusiastic joint range of motion by therapists, which leads to a hematoma and new bone formation in the young fibrous tissue; changes in O_2 and CO_2 exchange in the proximal blood circulation of paralyzed limbs; a reaction of perivascular connective tissue cells growing into injured tissue from surrounding areas; protein synthesis from degenerative muscle, which promotes ossification in local connective tissue cells; or some aberrant mucopolysaccharide metabolism that incurs ossification in connective tissue (Guttmann 1976; Guyton 1971). None of the theories has led to the specific identification of the precipitating factor necessary for the development of para-articular ossification.

Pierce and Nickel (1977) describe the histological characteristics as follows:

> The structural aspect of the PAO mass consists of a cortex about 1 mm thick, and a tightly latticed spongiosa which is less well-defined than in normal bone. It is lamellar with occasional Haversian systems that show features of new bone formation as in a fracture callus. The central part of the trabeculae is occasionally replaced by the remains of woven bone. There are a few osteoblasts and osteoclasts which indicate new bone formation, but not to a large extent. There is an occasional presence of microfractures of transverse orientation that are superimposed on already organized bone and are probably the reason for radionucleide uptake during the evolution of PAO. In places, the PAO bone is flanked by areas of edematous fibroblastic, osteogenic connective tissue which lines the grooves along the surface of the PAO as well as being associated with atrophic muscular fibers embedded in the bony mass. The connective tissue is without inflammatory infiltration. Microscopically, the newly formed bone consists of woven trabeculae undergoing osteoclastic erosion and the

beginning formation of a lamellar structure which demonstrates the usual characteristics of fibrillar ossification in progress.

Para-articular ossification may develop without any connection with muscle tissue, notable in aponeurotic tissue and in connective tissue. However, muscle fibers may be involved in long-standing PAO and may surround important blood vessels (D'Ambrosia 1977). Since osteoblasts secrete large quantities of alkaline phosphatase when they are active in the formation of new bone matrix and the alkaline phosphatase is diffused into the bloodstream, the level of alkaline phosphatase can be used as a measurement of new bone formation (Guyton 1971). Most investigators agree that the alkaline phosphatase blood level is more reliable than the serum phosphorus, even though both values are increased due to the bone and calcium metabolism involved in bone remodeling.

PSYCHOSOCIAL COMPONENTS AND THE IMPACT OF DIAGNOSIS

In the previous discussion, it was noted that PAO most often occurs during the first four months post-injury and usually involves the 25- to 40-year-old individual. This has tremendous implications for the spinal cord–injured patient, for this is the time when he is attempting to adjust to the trauma of the disability as well as to the changing self-concept that the injury invokes. Depending on the stage of his coping, the addition of a new entity, that of decreased movement secondary to para-articular ossification or at least the appearance of para-articular ossification on the X-ray, adds another factor to cope with in the ever-evolving adjustment process. Experience has shown that the more severe the loss in terms of disruption of total personality functioning, the more intense will be the reaction to the new occurrence of PAO (Hohmann 1975). Depending on the phase of the patient's reaction, one may see increased anger, depression, denial, withdrawal, or increased dependence. The patient may have begun to see some positive aspects of the rehabilitation program despite his disabilities. With the development of PAO, he is likely to become frustrated and feel that further cooperation in the program is futile. This is also illustrated by the fact that when there is a loss, grieving must occur. If the patient is already grieving for multiple sensory, motor, and body image problems, the addition of a new pathology adds an extra burden. During this time, a great strain is often placed on family members or significant others. They may feel guilty, useless, or hostile in attempting to deal with the patient's spinal cord injury as well as the diagnosis of PAO. Frequently, because of their misunderstanding, they will make demands for new treatment or discourage the continuance of the rehabilitation program. Family members, especially if the patient is young and living at home, may promote greater dependency and further the patient's reaction of depression, internalized hostility, or withdrawal. There may be an increased incentive for married individuals to dissociate themselves from the family because of a feeling of uselessness and a decreased self-concept. Often they will insist upon a divorce (Hohmann 1975; Stewart 1978).

Another aspect of psychological impact is the feeling of staff who are caring for the patient. Because such staff cannot see the ossification unless it is far advanced, they tend to minimize the patient's complaints. This further enhances the feelings of frustration and anger on the patient's part.

The best approach for all concerned is one of support through daily explanations of what is happening as a result of the disease process. It is also important to explain the results of lab work and X-rays as well as to allow the patient to express fears and anger. This is the time when family members should be involved in the daily care of the patient and be helped to understand the necessity for exercise, turning, position changes, and frequent lab work, X-rays, and bone scans.

A therapeutic program that fosters rehabilitation teaches independence through learning self-help skills for daily living. A daily exercise program is an integral part of the program. Such rehabilitation programs are designed to diminish the medical, social, psychological, economic, and vocational impact of the spinal cord injury. Therapy may not progress as rapidly for the patient with PAO as for other patients with the same level of cord lesion. Thus, the patient may need help to set realistic goals that he or she can hope to accomplish.

SUBJECTIVE DATA

Since the SCI patient will not experience pain, most subjective data comes from the history of the spinal cord injury and joint swelling below the level of injury. Heat and erythema usually accompany the swelling, and the swelling may extend to the entire extremity. Limitation of motion is present.

Other conditions can present the same or similar picture, and must be ruled out by history and/or appropriate testing. Conditions to rule out are septic arthritis, gout, bone tumor, osteoporosis, metabolic disorders, collagen or autoimmune disorders, and renal or prostatic disease. These disorders not only may present with the same symptoms, but they also cause similar variations in serum calcium, phosphorus, and alkaline phosphatase and signs of inflammation.

OBJECTIVE DATA

Laboratory, X-ray, and nuclear findings are incorporated into determination of the stage of the disorder. Stages listed by Nicholas (1973) and Tibone et al. (1978) are:

Stage I: Soft tissue swelling, elevated serum alkaline phosphatase, negative X-ray, and positive bone scan.

Stage II: Soft tissue swelling, elevated serum alkaline phosphatase, positive X-ray findings, and positive bone scan.

Stage III: Elevated serum alkaline phosphatase, positive X-ray findings, and positive bone scan.

Stage IV: Positive X-ray findings with decreasing activity on bone scan.

The time period between each stage is variable, and findings will vary depending on the length of time from initial injury when the patient was first evaluated. Initial evaluation should include:

1. Muscle and sensory examination to determine the level of neurological deficit. Para-articular ossification, when present, always involves joints below the level of the spinal cord injury.
2. Range of joint mobility determination.
3. Inspection for localized swelling, heat, pain, and redness of a joint and extremity. These symptoms often occur early in the process and precede roentgenographic changes by several weeks. Such symptoms usually disappear after four to ten weeks. The most common sites affected are points anterior to the hip and the medial aspect of the knee. If the patient has sensory sparing, pain will occur first. If there is complete cord transection, there will only be restriction of motion.
4. AP and lateral X-ray of the joint or joints involved. The appearance of immature para-articular ossification is characterized by "the absence of a distinct margin separating the ossified tissue from the surrounding soft tissue and the absence of linear trabeculations" (Pierce and Nickel 1977). As the disorder progresses, the bone gradually becomes trabeculated and mature throughout.
5. Serum alkaline phosphatase: In most labs the normal reading is between 30 to 115 mg/ml. Usually elevated early in the course of the disease and will remain so from six to eight months (Pierce and Nickel 1977). Any slight elevation is considered to be a contraindication to surgical treatment because of the active osteogenic process.
6. Bone scan is a useful parameter only if serum findings are available. These findings are necessary to determine the maturity of the para-articular ossification. It is a more sensitive indicator of osteoblastic activity than the alkaline phosphatase test. However, in the read-out, the anterior superior iliac spine cannot always be used as a comparison marker because if there is a large amount of ectopic bone, it will extend over that landmark (Tibone et al. 1978).
7. Laboratory tests to rule out other disease processes.
    a. Complete blood count with differential. This test would be done to rule out any evidence of blood dyscrasias, sepsis or thrombophlebitis that could precipitate similar symptoms to PAO.

b. Sedimentation rate. This test would assist in ruling out an infectious process, joint disease, or significant tissue necrosis.

c. SMA 6 and 12—with special emphasis on calcium, phosphorus, uric acid, glucose, sodium, BUN, and albumin. These values would help to rule out a metabolic disorder such as hyperthyroidism, hyperparathyroidism, gout, arthritis, and renal disease. These values also would be affected by a thrombo-embolic episode.

Electrocardiogram (EKG) is done to rule out cardiac involvement, which can result from metabolic or renal disease.

Follow-up tests usually include a monthly serum alkaline phosphatase and a bone scan. Since at least 14 to 18 months are needed for the ossification process to reach maturity, it is most important that both parameters be followed to determine the most opportune time for surgery, if it is indicated. If the bone scan is grossly abnormal or if there is a sudden increase in the alkaline phosphatase, the physician should be contacted immediately.

TREATMENT PLAN

INITIAL PLAN

1. Obtain a physical therapy consult for gentle, passive range of motion to the affected joint and active range of motion to other extremities. It is important to remember that loss of mineral from bone occurs more rapidly when the bone is non-utilized. Maintenance of function (even passive) decreases further mineral loss that might contribute to PAO.

2. Encourage and/or provide meticulous attention to skin and positioning to avoid decubitus ulcers and other joint contractures.

3. Encourage a well-balanced diet with adequate intake of calcium and vitamin D. Fluid intake should be at least 4,000 cc per day to decrease the effects of immobilization on protein synthesis and renal unction and to minimize the effects of the osteoclastic activity on other bony growth.

4. Administer Didronel (etidronate disodium) when prescribed to inhibit bone resportion and bone formation. The drug acts by modifying the crystal growth of calcium hydroxyapatite by chemisorption onto the crystal surface. It has been found to reduce the incidence of heterotropic bone formation as well as to retard the progression of immature masses. Didronel cannot dissolve already formed masses, but it appears to restrict the severity of the clinical manifestations of restriction of movement. Indocin (brand name; generic—Indomethacin) therapy may be used as an alternative as well as X-ray therapy.

SURGICAL INTERVENTION

Surgery is considered when there are less than 50 degrees of hip flexion or if there is total immobility of a joint with increased pain. The timing of surgery is important for two reasons: (a) Removal of ectopic bone too early may result in further ossification and hematoma formation. (b) If the surgery is too late, the new bone may be extremely hard and envelop such important vessels as the femoral vein or artery.

The risks of surgery need to be weighed against the expected benefits. The major risk is hematoma formation that may progress to wound break-down, infection, sinus formation, and even osteomyelitis. Surgical management generally includes:

1. Broad spectrum antibiotic coverage. Keflex, 2 gm I.V. every six hours, is usually started two days pre-operatively and continued until the seventh post-operative day.
2. Suction drainage of the wounds either by Hemovac or Jackson-Pratt.
3. If the hip is the operated area, the patient is then maintained with his hip and knee flexed 90 degrees to decrease the dead space available for hematoma accumulation (Wharton and Morgan 1970).
4. Careful attention to skin care to decrease decubitus ulcer formation.
5. Didronel (etidronate disodium) should be started at 20 mg/Kg/day for two weeks prior to surgery and continued at 10 mg/Kg/day for 39 weeks post-operatively. There is evidence that such a regime will delay post-operative recurrence of PAO (Guttmann 1976; Stover et al. 1976).

PATIENT/FAMILY EDUCATION

1. During the initial stage, the patient and family members or significant others must be taught about the disease process and the importance of the various X-ray, lab, and nuclear medicine tests.
2. A home exercise program can be developed and taught to family members or a trained attendant.
3. The patient, if seen as an outpatient, must understand the necessity for continued follow-up to determine the maturity of the ossification.
4. When surgery is indicated, the patient and his family should receive an explanation of the operative procedure, risks, and a description of the positioning so that discomfort and worry can be minimized in the post-operative period. Once the incision is healed, the patient and his family need to understand and learn:
   a. the exercise program
   b. bowel and bladder care

c. skin care
d. the importance of continuing to take the Didronel, and which side effects can be managed and which need to be reported
e. the importance of continued follow-up care to check for any recurrence of the para-articular ossification.

12

Secondary Amyloidosis

ISABELLE HOLLIS and ALICE McROY

Although amyloidosis occurs only infrequently in the general population, it is a disease that was first described over 130 years ago and was named by Virchow in 1853. The term "amyloid" was applied to the extracellular fibrous deposits because of the starchlike characteristics of iodine staining. For many years amyloid was thought to be a carbohydrate. More recently, however, amyloid has been identified histologically as a protein consisting of polypeptide chains (Glenner et al. 1973). Although the natural history of this disease is still poorly understood today, amyloidosis is defined as extracellular deposition of the fibrous protein amyloid in one or more sites in the body (Isselbacher et al. 1980). This complex disease may involve virtually any organ system and result in the subsequent destruction of vital organs, or may cause few clinical consequences, depending on the site of deposition. The following classification of amyloidosis illustrates the complexities involved in this disease entity:

1. primary amyloidosis with no evidence of pre-existing or co-existing disease
2. amyloid associated with multiple myeloma
3. secondary amyloidosis associated with chronic infection or inflammatory diseases
4. heredofamilial amyloidosis
5. local amyloidosis (no systemic involvement)
6. amyloidosis associated with aging (Isselbacher et al. 1980; van Rijswijk and Van Heusden 1979).

The focus of this chapter will be on secondary amyloidosis, with specific interest in amyloidosis occurring as a complication of paralysis resulting from traumatic spinal cord injury. Secondary amyloidosis has long been associated with a number of common chronic diseases that are characterized by long-term infection and/or inflammation, autoimmune diseases, and conditions in which there is excessive tissue breakdown and wasting (Anderson and Kissane 1977). Among the diseases that have been associated with secondary amyloidosis are chronic tuberculosis, osteomyelitis, lupus erythematosis, rheumatoid arthritis, colitis, syphilis, ankylosing spondylitis, and leprosy. Terms applied to secondary amyloidosis are typical, genuine, visceral, and general parenchymatous (Briggs 1961). Several authors have reported on the incidence of secondary amyloidosis as a complication of paraplegia. Among the cord-injured population, it is linked primarily with chronic pressure sores and underlying osteomyelitis and is accompanied by a high incidence of severe renal involvement (Tribe and Silver 1969; Comarr 1958).

INCIDENCE, EPIDEMIOLOGY, AND ETIOLOGY

A review of the literature reveals varying estimates of the rate of occurrence of secondary amyloidosis in paraplegics. Tribe and Silver (1969) predicted that "up to 5 percent of all paraplegics develop amyloidosis from the septic complications of spinal paralysis." During the past several decades, the prevalence of many infectious and inflammatory diseases has declined due to the proliferation of antibiotics and specific chemotherapy for many of the chronic diseases. In addition, improved surgical techniques have shortened the course of some of the chronic diseases that heretofore were frequently complicated by secondary amyloidosis. Therefore, there has been a decline in secondary amyloidosis associated with diseases such as tuberculosis, syphilis, leprosy, and other diseases considered suppurative (Robbins and Cotran 1979).

Coincidently, improved medical care, antibiotics, and sophisticated techniques have prolonged the lives of the spinal cord–injured and thereby increased the prevalence of secondary complications, including amyloidosis. Although amyloidosis was associated with paralysis as early as 1876, there are few references in the literature before World War II because paraplegics usually died before they could develop amyloidosis (Tribe and Silver 1969). Now, the spinal cord–injured individual has nearly a normal life expectancy, so amyloidosis more frequently complicates the health picture. Approximately ten thousand new spinal cord injuries occur per annum in the United States, with the percentage of quadriplegics increasing steadily. It is felt that the incidence of secondary amyloidosis is higher in quadriplegics than paraplegics.

The chief causative factor of amyloidosis secondary to paraplegia is decubitus ulceration associated with underlying osteomyelitis. These patients respond poorly to therapy and require various skin grafts, which frequently break down to form indolent ulcers. The incidence of osteomyelitis is not easy to assess but is important in etiological considerations. When amyloidosis occurs in the cord–injured without pressure sores, it is thought to be the result of chronic urinary tract infection with the formation of pus.

The neurogenic bladder frequently requires an indwelling catheter, which causes irritation and subsequent pus-forming infection that predisposes to an ascending pyelonephritis. When chronic pyelonephritis is accompanied by hypomotility of the ureters, secondary to neurogenic dysfunction and prolonged bedrest with secondary hypercalcemia, then formation of renal calculi may follow (Berkow 1978).

Tribe and Silver described the etiology of amyloidosis in chronic paralysis leading to ultimate death from renal failure as a dichotomy. On one hand, the development of pressure sores leads to osteomyelitis, which then gives rise to amyloidosis and eventual renal failure (1969). As the increased population of SCI persons grows older, the results of prolonged malnutrition, electrolyte imbalance (particularly nitrogen imbalance with lowered serum proteins) and chronic infections are being seen. These three conditions—malnutrition, electrolyte imbalance, and infection—when prolonged are the precursors of the development of secondary amyloidosis.

PATHOPHYSIOLOGY

Amyloidosis is a disturbance of endogenous protein metabolism, either primary or as a result of chronic suppuration or tissue breakdown. Deposition of amyloid is either general or local, causing organic dysfunction. Amyloid is a protein complex having starchlike characteristics produced and deposited in tissues during certain pathological states. The protein polypeptide chain that comprises the amyloid deposits is arranged in beta-pleated sheet configuration, resulting in resistance to proteolytic digestion. The fibrils are insoluble under physiologic conditions (Anderson and Kissane 1977). They stain readily with eosin dyes, are without definite structure, and are crystalline, glassy, and translucent. They are distributed throughout the body, and are homogenous and highly refractile. The accumulation of this fibrilar glycoprotein amyloid may be in amounts sufficient to impair normal function in the tissue. No organ system is entirely exempt from amyloid deposits, but involvement of the central nervous system is rare.

Although the basic cause or defect is still unknown, the disorder seems to be the abnormal physiological nature of the secretions of the exocrine glands. Pathologic changes are present in organs containing mucus-secreting glands, such as the liver, lungs, pancreas, and submaxillary glands (Baum 1974). It has been suggested (Robbins 1979) that "amyloidosis is an expression of some derangement in immunoregulatory controls, possibly the induction of immune tolerance following protracted antigenic challenge." Once amyloid has been produced and deposited in the tissues, its affinity for Congo red dye can be seen both in vivo and in prepared tissues. It is made up primarily of a well-defined fibril, distinct from other extracellular structural proteins, which occurs in two forms. One has an N-terminal sequence that is homologous with a portion of the variable region of an immunoglobulin light chain; the other has a unique N-terminal sequence of a non-immunoglobulin protein called "AA" protein (Berkow 1978).

Organs containing amyloid deposits have been described as being waxy, as having a firm rubbery consistency, and as being pink or gray in color. Hypertrophy of organs, particularly the liver, spleen, heart, and kidney, are not uncommon (Isselbacher et al. 1980). Although amyloid usually involves several vital organs, functional disturbance in paraplegics is primarily seen in the kidney, resulting in chronic renal failure and eventual death. The nonbranching, rigid fibrils of amyloid are frequently laid down first in the mesangial cells of the kidney and Kupffer cells of the liver. The amyloid deposits in the kidney are chiefly in the glomeruli but may also involve the renal arterioles and peri-tubular tissue. In many instances, pyelonephritis is also present. Although kidneys may have amyloidosis, acute pyelonephritis may occur as the terminal event and vice versa. Amyloid may also be deposited in local masses in the kidney (Tribe and Silver 1969).

PSYCHOSOCIAL ASPECTS

The person's self-image, adjustment to the original injury, and acceptance by the family are all deciding factors in the manner of coping with an additional stressful situation. The individual who makes a poor adjustment to the injury frequently experiences repeated, serious pressure sores, with long hospitalization as a result. Nurses may begin to stereotype and categorize patients, especially in the situation where long-term care is required, such as for the cord injured. The most common response individuals feel when they perceive dehumanization is anger (Travelbee 1966). The poorly adjusted individual frequently exhibits anger, frustration, depression, and low self-esteem. Travis (1961) stated that the "lives of most paraplegics are burdensome, frustrating, and physiologically complex."

To a large extent, the ability of patients discharged from the hospital to cope with an additional serious illness is determined by their status in the family. The single young adult male may have difficulty accepting an additional disability. There is the original injury with an unfavorable outcome that he is attempting to accept. He occupies a peripheral family role and is not part of a stable family. He is ill-prepared for a major readjustment in his life situation, and this diagnosis represents a catastrophic event (Dinsdale et al. 1971). He has to learn to cope with a radically changed life situation, loss of self-esteem and "maleness." There may be a pronounced dependency-independency conflict. Early mobilization of any family and community resources will assist this patient by alleviating social and financial problems so that he can devote his energies to a plan of action and care that may arrest the amyloidosis.

The married male has different needs. He occupies a central role in the family, has a better premorbid adjustment, and has had more educational and vocational training. He has a stable location and more community support. Illness is accepted better, hospital management is not a problem, and the patient either returns to his previous vocation or is trained to a different but suitable one. The main problem is one of role reversal. If he is unable to earn as before and cannot share fully with household tasks, he is more dependent on his wife and children. His needs dictate a family therapy approach to problems raised by role reversal. The whole family must be involved in therapy and their healthy resources used to reduce role conflict (Dinsdale et al. 1971). Any premorbid marital or family problems must be examined, and attention must be directed to effective communication, problem solving, constructive expression of feelings, and promotion of closeness. The family should be involved prior to admission since the patient already has a cord injury. With the diagnosis of amyloidosis, it would be helpful to have the family remain intensively involved in all stages of treatment. The community support system could and should be used to assist the family.

The married female patient does not undergo a pronounced role reversal and is better able to adjust to her chosen role. She can still function as wife and mother as well as a professional. The problems usually center around acceptance of her disability, the need for more task sharing on the part of other family members, and consideration of architectural changes in the home and at work to assist with the completion of tasks. With the spouse, consideration has to be given to a group approach to deal with the exploration and reduction of sexual problems and concerns.

Just as the patient adjusts to his injury and illness, so must the family go through the completed process of understanding, accepting and adjusting. At first there may be grief. There may be no visible progress, and the family has to live with knowledge that the condition could be terminal. Interwoven into the family's feelings may be a repressed wish that the person would die and prevent the pain and frustration that is ahead. Then rationalization sets in and the illness and its accompaniments are accepted. At this point, the significant others can begin helping the patient (Garfield 1979).

The patient may be verbally abusive or assaultive. Relatives could have a difficult time deciding if this behavior represents his true feelings. The patient may become complaining, demanding and dependent, and the family confused and angry by demands that seem out of character. The relatives may become angry when the patient does not credit them for their efforts. A feeling of helpless frustration may persist.

Sometimes the family may carry an additional burden because of the feeling of contributing to or causing the accident in which the patient was originally injured. Decubitus ulcers may have been allowed to progress to large, dirty, necrotic pressure sores, and the family may harbor guilt because adequate care was not given. Even when relatives had nothing to do with the injury or condition, some feel guilty. They feel they should have foreseen the possibility of the original accident and taken steps to prevent it, thereby preventing the complication of amyloidosis. Eventually these guilt feelings are rationalized as a method of relieving responsibility. Families often suffer a significant financial expense. If the patient is no longer able to work or has limited income, the family's standard of living could be affected (Dinsdale et al. 1971). The need for a humanistic, emphatic approach to the spinal cord injured is evident.

SUBJECTIVE AND OBJECTIVE DATA

Diagnosis

Characteristic symptoms or signs of amyloidosis are lacking. Clinical manifestations are nonspecific and usually originate in the organ or system affected. Often they are obscured by the underlying disease, which may be fatal before secondary amyloidosis is suspected. Since the symptoms may resemble those of a variety of other disorders, amyloidosis must frequently be considered in the differential diagnosis. Although widespread amyloid infiltration may be present, clinical evidence of organ dysfunction is most frequently related to renal failure, with gastrointestinal and liver involvement less frequently the responsible sites. Subjective symptoms may include light-headedness or syncope; reports of gastrointestinal disturbances of anorexia, hemorrhage, or chronic diarrhea; reports of weight loss; or reports of hair loss.

Objective signs may include:

1. *The nephrotic syndrome* is the most striking manifestation. In the early stages only slight proteinuria may be noted. Protein loss in the urine of more than 5 gms in 24 hours is suggestive of renal amyloidosis. Later the distinctive symptom complex develops with anasarca, hypoproteinemia, and massive proteinuria. The urine sediment often contains RBCs. The creatinine clearance is low, and metabolic acidosis is frequently present. BUN is elevated.
2. *Hepatomegaly* may occur if the disease is in the liver. Jaundice is rare. Portal hypertension may occur with esophageal varices and ascites.

Splenomegaly may also be present in advanced disease. Lab tests show low BSP excretion, elevated serum alkaline phosphatase, and decreased serum albumin.

3. *Skin lesions* may be waxy or translucent. Purpura may result from amyloidosis of small cutaneous vessels. Petechiae or ecchymosis may develop spontaneously or upon mild trauma (gentle stroking of the skin). Papules are the classic and most characteristic cutaneous manifestation. They are smooth, shiny, waxy, and vary in color depending on the extent and duration of local hemorrhage. They are non-tender and, if deposited on the eyelids, may cause the patient to seek help for cosmetic reasons. Location is generally about the body folds, but any area can be involved (Rubinow and Cohen 1978).

4. Other patients present with thick, firm, smooth, tight skin resembling scleroderma. Usually the face, neck, and hands are involved. Facial involvement results in loss of wrinkles and a fixed, rigid, expressionless face. The insidious tightening of the skin may cause progressive flexion contractures and restriction of motion of the joints in the hand (Rubinow and Cohen 1978).

5. *Alopecia* may be a striking clinical feature. Hair loss is usually patchy and confined to the scalp.

6. *Nodules, tumors* or plaques, skin tags, or bullous formations may present.

7. *Cardiac involvement* may be manifest as intractable heart failure or any of the common arhythmias.

8. *Hemorrhage* includes atrial standstill (Berkow 1978) and malabsorption in the bowel. Steatorrhea may be present. Serum carotene may be abnormal.

9. *Thyroid involvement* may present with firm, symmetric, nontender goiter.

10. *Arthropathy* may mimic rheumatoid arthritis.

11. *Peripheral neuropathy.*

12. Other signs include waxy casts in urine, macroglossia, hypertension and fluid in the serous cavities. Blood shows anemia, elevated sedimentation rate, and white count greater than $12,000/c \times mm$.

SPECIAL DIAGNOSTIC TESTS

Definite diagnosis of secondary amyloidosis can be made only by viewing biopsied tissue which has been stained with Congo red. When viewed by polarized microscopy, a characteristic green birefringence is seen (Tribe and Silver 1969). A method to differentiate between primary and secondary amyloidosis is to first stain the tissue sample with potassium permanganate. If the tissue then loses sensitivity to Congo red, it is not amyloid, a protein that is found in secondary amyloidosis (van Rijswijk 1979).

The most widely accepted method of obtaining tissue for diagnostic tests is rectal biopsy. Different authors rate the accuracy of this test from 75 percent to 90 percent. Amyloid deposits are usually found in the submucosal layer. Gingival biopsies as well as peroral jejuneum biopsies have been used. Kidney or liver biopsies are also about 90 percent accurate, but considered dangerous because of the possibility of hemorrhage (Stanbury et al.1978). Skin biopsies can be taken from the site of plaque formation. A new diagnostic method is the needle biopsy of subcutaneous fat. This is considered at least as accurate as the rectal biopsy and more convenient. Since operative procedures of the kidneys may be done from time to time in the SCI patient, it is recommended that tissue specimens routinely be analyzed for amyloidosis (Stanbury et al. 1978).

MANAGEMENT

There is no cure for secondary amyloidosis. The control of the underlying infectious and/or inflammatory disease is imperative. Some authors report a regression of amyloid deposits when the infectious disease is eliminated or controlled (Triger and Joekes 1973). Early, vigorous control of hypertension is recommended as well as correction of abnormal electrolyte levels.

Amyloid nephrosis may respond to diuretics and intensive protein replacement therapy. However, renal failure may have progressed to the point of needing dialysis by the time the patient presents himself. At the present time paraplegics and quadriplegics are not generally considered as candidates for renal transplants.

As long as large amounts of protein are being lost via urine or pressure sores, protein replacement is necessary. Blood transfusions are sometimes required. Meticulous attention should be given to the patient's nutritional status. High caloric, high protein diets with vitamin supplements including ascorbic acid and liver extract are usually recommended.

Most authorities agree that the best treatment is prevention. Maintaining the patient in a catheter-free state, free as possible from urinary tract infections, with free drainage of urine without high residuals is extremely important. All other foci of infection must also be controlled, such as pressure sores and osteomyelitis. In patients with deep and infected ulcers around a joint, particularly the hip or knee, early closure with some sort of skin graft or flap is of great importance. When there is severe spasm, with or without contractures, that would interfere with or prevent the healing of a plastic procedure, it may be necessary to do an anterior rhizotomy or subarachnoid alcohol block before doing the plastic surgery. Relief of spasms is temporarily obtained by the use of antispasmodic drugs such as Baclofen, Dantrium, or Valium. Antibiotics are given to control the infection. The ulcer is drained and cleansed several times daily with a strong agent such as Betadine and sterile protective dressings applied. Whether adrenocortical steroids are helpful is questionable (Stanbur et al. 1978).

PATIENT EDUCATION

Patient teaching is an integral part of nursing for the spinal cord injured. Specifically, the patient should be taught meticulous skin care with prevention of pressure sores given paramount importance. Frequent position changes, use of mirror to inspect skin, keeping skin clean, dry and oiled, and active and passive range of motion exercises are cornerstones for prevention of skin breakdown. All patients and their significant others should know not only the cause and prevention of skin ulcers, but also what to do if any pressure area or skin insults do occur. Treating a superficial sore promptly minimizes the likelihood of underlying osteomyelitis.

The patient needs to be taught the importance of avoiding urinary problems by regular bladder care (using aseptic technique if intermittent catherization is required) and by forcing fluids. Regular check-up examinations are also important for prompt recognition of infection and early treatment.

The importance of a good high-protein diet needs to be stressed. The patient should know the reason for the vitamin supplements and be given information how to incorporate needed foods into a diet he finds palatable. The patient and his family should not be deprived of reasonable hope for the future. They need to know that for many patients, the course of amyloidosis may be prolonged and last many years, and that treatment of the underlying conditions will help in the remission of the disease (Kyle and Bayrd 1975). In periods of remission, the patient will be both clinically and subjectively improved.

Appendix

STAGES OF PSYCHOSOCIAL ADJUSTMENT
FOLLOWING A SPINAL CORD INJURY

HELEN PAUTSCH

Patient Behavior	Therapeutic Approach
A. SHOCK	
• Emotional paralysis or numbness, similar to affect of patient following seizure of E.S.T.—as if a "fuse blew."	Support and presence of significant others.
• Reality perception is sharp. Person knows something has happened but emotional response is blocked out or "frozen."	Feelings and touch are more appropriate than words.
• Thinking and behavior are remote, automatic, and mechanical—apart from person, "depersonalized."	Do not give details of prognosis since it won't be recalled later.
• Anxiety level is low because of protective emotional paralysis. Shock serves to insulate patient from the reality.	
Time 3 days to 2 weeks.	
B. REALIZATION	
• Numbness of shock phase replaced by recognition of the threat to self-preservation, which leads to overwhelming anxiety, panic, and feelings of helplessness.	Communicate to patient and family that they are not alone.
• Overcome by disability.	Let patient know others are available to help and that their response will be reliable, predictable, and honest.

- Panic, screaming, and crying. May seem withdrawn or disoriented. May be irritable, have sleep irregularities.
- Not conscious of what's being done to him, "not available" psychologically.
- Can't think clearly, unable to plan.

Allow patient to set pace for discussion of disability. Both shock and realization may be fleeting because anxiety is so intense they can't be maintained without total psychic disorganization.

Protect patient from harm during periods of panic.

C. DEFENSIVE RETREAT

- A variety of behaviors that serve to protect patient from painful reality. Behavior of the individual is influenced by his/her pre-injury defense mechanisms.

1. *Denial-Disbelief*

- Behavior that says, "There's nothing wrong with me."

Recognize patient's need to have a defense mechanism and the function it serves.

- Failure to acknowledge reality ("I will walk").

Accept how patient says he is.

- May claim something else in order to decrease threat ("I'm incomplete").

Convey understanding of what patient says ("I know how much you want to walk") but do not support the patient in his behavior to avoid treatment.

- Avoids reality by "forgetting" to follow instructions, missing therapy appointments, and withdrawing.
- Refuses to do required tasks.

Set limits on behavior, but do not stress the permanence of his disability, since this may intensify denial.

- May try to control treatment by developing other symptoms.
- May act as if nothing has happened—may be happy-go-lucky.

Recognize patient may not be aware of his denial; what he says is what he believes is true.

2. *Intellectualization-Rationalization*

- "I can think about it but not feel it."

Listen.

- Patient talks freely about injury with little expression of feeling.

Attempt to help patient express how he feels.

- Can say "I know I'm paralyzed and I've accepted it."
- Patients talks and talks but doesn't cry.

"It must be unbearable to think about . . "

Convey attitude of acceptance of feelings: "It's okay to cry."

- Often wants extensive details about nervous system, surgery, or specifics of treatment plans.

- May have explanation (rationalization) for circumstances without *emotion.*

3. *Anger (Projection)*

- Projects responsibility for injury and cure, often accusing personnel of bad treatment.
- Hostile toward staff who make him aware of limitations/dependency.

Recognize patient is angry at the injury and don't take anger expressed at you personally.
Let patient verbalize anger, acknowledging his right to feel as he does. "It must be frustrating for you to . . .".

- Cynicism or provocative, bossing behavior, "What did I do to deserve this?"

Don't attempt to defend staff to the patient.

4. *Regression*

- Return to earlier forms of behavior.
- May become as helpless as a child or have temper tantrums.
- May withdraw, give up.

Do not accept the role of a parent. Maintain the attitude that you are there to help him help himself.
Support independence in behavior and decision making. Talk through activities to be done, giving patient small choices to make such as color of socks, station on radio.

- Dependency because of injury may trigger regression to more infantile behavior.
- Defensive retreat may last for weeks, months, years; some never escape it completely.

Express confidence that patient will gradually be able to exert more control over behavior.

D. ACKNOWLEDGMENT

- The real work of adjustment.
- Developing awareness of what has happened and its implications.
- Reality begins to break through defenses.
- Recognizes dependency and may become irritable and impatient or apathetic and withdrawn.
- Expresses *feelings* regarding disability vs. intellectual statements. Expressions may be self-depreciatory: "I'm not as good as before."
- Mourns loss of function, opportunities, and "old self."

Provide supportive presence and a listening ear.
Let patient work it through by expressing feelings and grieving over loss.
Encourage patient to express feelings regarding the future.

Identify the patient's assets that can be strengths to help work through his disability.

Support positive validation of the person.

Allow patient to progress at his/her own rate.

- Anxiety may be near panic and suicide may be a possibility.

Psychotherapy is most useful in this stage to help the patient acquire new motivation, new interest, and progress to making realistic life plans.

E. COPING

- Sometimes referred to as adaptation or acceptance.
- Coping suggests "I'm trying to make the best of it."
- Reintegration of concept of self to include the disability.
- Pursues positive goals within potential: "I am not, nor ever will, be quite the same person, but basically I am still me and there are ways I can be of value to the world around me."
- Tests reality as it now is. Reorganizes life according to present resources.
- Satisfying experiences increase.

Help patient develop realistic plans.

Expose patient to resources; teach problem-solving.

Provide full support via growth-oriented or vocational counseling.

Don't expect unrealistic progress, since patient's success in coping will be correlated with prior personality and support systems.

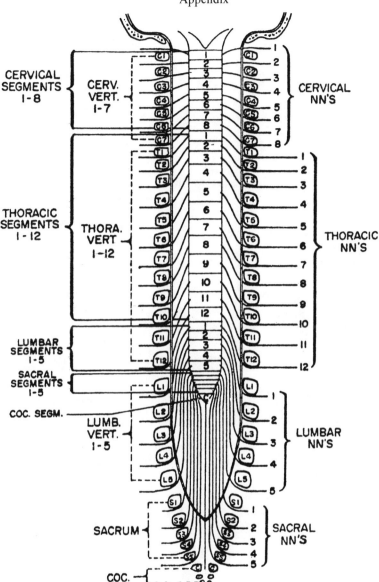

Figure A.1 The spinal cord is that part of the central nervous axis lodged in the bony vertebral column. There are afferent (sensory) nerves and efferent (motor) nerves exiting on each side of the spinal segments. The cord consists of eight cervical segments, 12 thoracic segments, 5 lumbar segments, 5 sacral segments, and 1 coccygeal segment. The cord ends at approximately L1–L2 level, but the nerves continue downward, exiting through corresponding vertebral openings, and begin to resemble "a horse's tail," thus being labeled the cauda equina. The conus medullaris is located at the upper lumbar segments where the cauda equina begins.

REFLEX   ARC

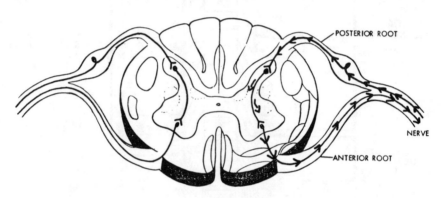

Figure A.2 Reflex activity in a reflex arc is defined as an impulse that travels inward over an afferent (sensory) pathway where it by-passes the brain, and synapses with innuncial cells which then send impulses through the efferent (motor) pathways outward to the periphery muscle, or organ.

REFLEXES

Definition: Reflected involuntary actions or movements elicited by a stimulus.

Cord Segment	Tendon Reflex	Normal Response	Remarks
C3, C4: Shoulder area	No demonstrative reflex elicited		There may be a partial or complete paresis of the diaphragm with a C3 lesion anteriorly, or a C4 lesion posteriorly.
C5, C6: Biceps and deltoid, radial side of arm down, including thumb and index finger	Biceps	Contraction of the biceps muscle when tendon is tapped.	When absent, indicates flaccid paralysis or paresis (lower motor neuron lesion). If hyperactive, indicative of spasticity of an upper motor neuron lesion.
C7, C8: Posterio-lateral aspect of arm from C6, including— ring, middle and little fingers	Triceps	Extension of the forearm when triceps tendon is tapped at the elbow, while the forearm hangs limp at right angle to the arm.	Abnormal when absent, indicating flaccid paralysis or paresis. Must be distinquished from carpal tunnel syndrome as opposed to lower motor neuron lesion.
L3, L4: From Greater Trochanter front and medial aspect of thigh and knee, over patella to median border of foot	Patellar	Contraction of quadraceps produced by sharply striking the ligamentus patellae when the leg hangs loosely flexed at right angle.	Abnormal when absent diminished. Indicates lower motor neuron lesion or flaccid paralysis. If hyperactive, denotes spasticity of upper motor neuron lesion.
L5: Anterio-Lateral Quadrant of leg to include great toe.	Post Tibial	Tapping of the tibia on the inner side of leg, either in homolateral adduction or crossed adduction from side to side, produces brisk response.	Response is absent or decreased in lower motor neuron lesions; hyperactive or spastic in upper motor neurons.
S1: Flexor aspect of thigh, over posterio-lateral quadrant of leg and lateral	Ankle	Contraction of the foot when tricep surae muscle is tapped.	Absence indicates paresis or paralysis of the peronei and tricep surae. Clonus is produced with pressure on the sole with dorso-

malleous, to include the 4th and 5th small toes.			flexion of the foot.
L5, S1: Dermatomes of L5 and S1 combination.	Babinski vs. Planter	Firm stroke along outer side of sole of foot from heel to base of 5th toe will produce normally a Planter response, which is a flexion of all toes.	Abnormal response is a Babinski, which produces dorsi-flexion of great toe and fanning out of other toes. Denotes Pyramidal Tract disease.
T7, L1: Intercostals and abdominal muscles, including the lower abdomen and pelvis.	Abdominal	Elicited by scratching or stroking abdominal skin. Normally the umbellicus moves toward point being stroked.	Absence may indicate pyramidal lesion, or it may be absent in older people, obese people, or in often, repeated pregnancies. It may also indicate direct damage to the reflex arc.
S4, S5: Penis and anal area.	Anal Reflex or Bulbo-cavernous	Contraction of the anal sphincter in response to pinching the glans at the base of penis or by tugging catheter.	This reflex if usually lost in cauda equinal lesions and results in flaccid paralysis.
L1, L2: Lower abdomen and hips.	Cremasteric	Evoked by stimulation or stroking front of inner side of upper thigh, resulting in the testes on the same side retracting or pulling up as the cremasteric muscle contracts.	Bilateral absence indicates upper motor neuron lesion or disease; unilateral absence, lower motor neuron involvement.

PRIORITY FUNCTIONAL LEVELS

Muscle	Dermatome Enervation
Deltoid and biceps	C5
Latissimus, serratus, pectoralis and radial wrist extensors	C6
Triceps, finger extensors and flexors	C7
Hand intrinsics, ulnar side of wrist and fingers	T1
Upper intercostals and upper back	T6
Abdominals and upper thoracics	T12
Hip flexors and quadraceps	L4

Despite considerable overlap in the dermatome chart and dermatome areas, the chart still remains an extremely helpful tool in evaluating and locating a spinal cord lesion and/or injury.

Figures A.3, A.4, and A.5 Dermatomes may be defined as areas of skin patterns that are supplied by afferent (sensory) nerve fibers which are useful in defining sensory nerve involvement in an illness or injury. Foerster is credited with labeling the following dermatome charts and is probably the one most commonly used.

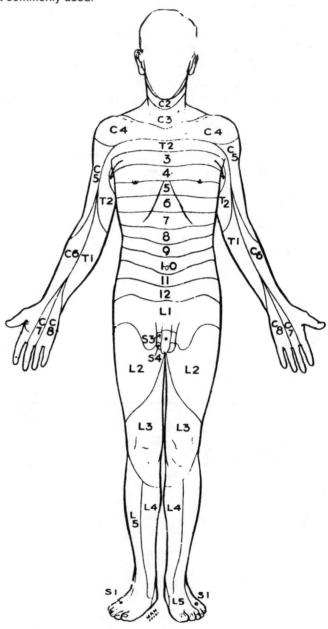

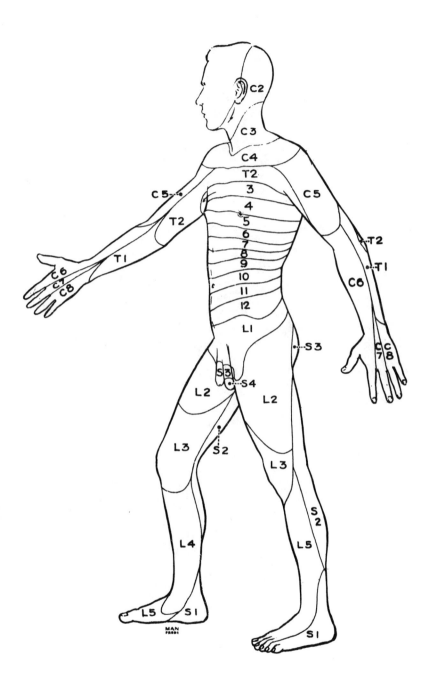

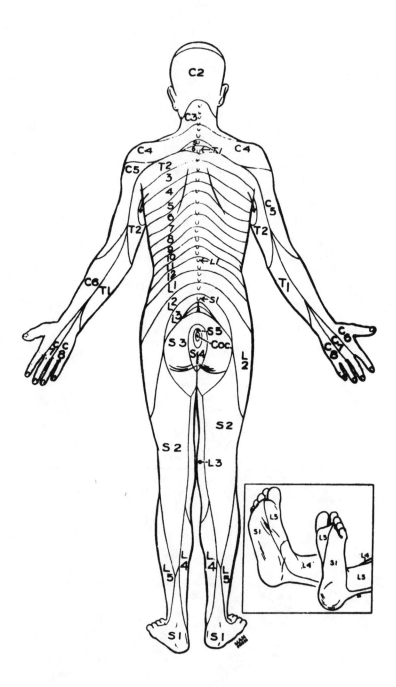

References

Anderson, T.P. 1977. "Psychosocial Factors Associated with Pressure Sores." *Archives of Physical Medicine and Rehabilitation* 60 (August): 341–45.

Anderson, W.A.D., and J.M. Kissane. 1977. *Pathology.* St. Louis: C.V. Mosby. Pp. 123–25.

Baker, Mary, E. Reyenos, et al. 1977. "Developing Strategies for Biofeedback." *Physical Therapy* 57 (April): 402–8.

Baum, G.L. 1974. *Textbook of Pulmonary Diseases.* 2nd edition. Boston: Little, Brown. Pp. 804–41, 930–31.

Beland, Irene. 1972. *Clinical Nursing: Pathophysiological and Psychosocial Approaches.* 2nd edition. London: The Macmillan Co.

Beland, Irene L., and Joyce Y. Passos. 1975. *Clinical Nursing.* New York: Macmillan.

Benvenuti, C. 1977. "Independence for the Paraplegic: The Bantam Respirator." *American Journal of Nursing.* May.

Berecek, Kathleen H. 1975. "Etiology of Decubitus Ulcers." *Nursing Clinics of North America* 10, no. 1: 157–70.

Berkow, R., ed. 1978. *The Merck Manual.* 13th edition. Rahway, N.J.: Merck, Sharp and Dohme Research Laboratory. Pp. 1241–42.

Bishop, Beverly. 1977. "Spasticity: Its Physiology and Management." *Physical Therapy* 57, no. 4 (April): 371–401.

Briggs, G.W. 1961. "Amyloidosis." *Annals of Internal Medicine* 55: 943–55.

Brooks, C., ed. 1979. *Integrative Functions of the Autonomic Nervous System.* Tokyo: University of Tokyo Press.

Bruckner, B.S., and L.P. Ince. 1977. "Biofeedback as an Experimental Treatment for Hypotension in a Patient with a Spinal Lesion." *Archives of Physical Medicine and Rehabilitation* 58 (February): 49–53.

Burke, David C. 1973. "Pain in Paraplegia." *Paraplegia* 10: 297–313.

Burke, David C., and D. Duncan Murray. 1975. *Handbook of Spinal Cord Medicine.* New York: Raven Press.

Carini, E., and G. Owens. 1978. *Neurological and Neuro Surgical Nursing.* St. Louis: C.V. Mosby.

Carter, R. 1979. "Medical Management of Pulmonary Complications of Spinal Cord Injured." In *Advances in Neurology*, Vol. 22, ed. R. Thompson and J. Green. New York: Raven Press.

Caslyn, Donald A., John Louks, and Charles W. Freeman. 1976. "The Use of the MMPI with Chronic Low Back Pain Patients with Mixed Diagnosis." *Journal of Clinical Psychology* 32, no. 3 (July): 532–36.

Chusid, J.G. 1976. *Correlative Neuroanatomy and Functional Neurology*. Los Altos, Calif.: Lange Medical Publications.

Chyatte, Samuel B. 1979. *Rehabilitation in Chronic Renal Failure*. Baltimore: Williams & Wilkins.

Clark, M.C. 19755. "Chest Pain." *Heart and Lung* 4, no. 6: 956–62.

Cole, T.M. 1979. "Sexuality and Physical Disabilities." *Archives of Sexual Behavior* 4, no. 4: 389–403.

Coleman, Pamela. 1976. "The Problem of Spasticity in the Management of the Spinal Cord–Injured Patient and Its Treatment, with Special Reference to Percutaneous Radiofrequency Thermal Selective Sensory Rhizotomy." *Journal of Neurosurgical Nursing* 8, no. 3: 97–103.

Comarr, A. Estin. 1977a. "Autonomic Dysreflexia." Pp. 181–85 in *The Total Care of Spinal Cord Injuries*, ed. D.S. Pierce and V.H. Nickel. Boston: Little, Brown.

———. 1977b. "Sexual Function in Patients with Spinal Cord Injury." Pp. 171–79 in Pierce and Nickel, ed., *The Total Care of Spinal Cord Injuries*.

———. 1979. "Urinary Bladder Disorders from Spinal Cord Injury." *Comprehensive Therapy* 9 (5 September): 37–46.

Comarr, A. Estin, and B. Gunderson. 1975. "Sexual Function in Traumatic Paraplegia and Quadriplegia." *American Journal of Nursing* (February): 250–55.

Cook, W.A., and L.R. King. 1979. "Vesicoureteral Reflux." In *Campbell's Urology*, Vol. 2, ed. J.H. Harrison, R. Gittes, and A. Perlmutter. 4th edition. Philadephia: W.B. Saunders.

Coon, W.W. 1974. "Operative Therapy of Venous Thromboembolism." *Modern Concepts of Cardiovascular Disease* 43, no. 2 (February): 71–75

Cressy, J., and A.E. Comarr. 1981. "Sexuality and Spinal Cord Injury." *Science Digest: Model Systems* 3: 23–30.

D'Agostino, J., and P. Welch. 1979. "The Phrenic Pacemaker." *Nursing 79* 9, no. 5.

Daly, C.R., and E.A. Kelly. 1972. "Prevention of Pulmonary Emboli: Intra-Caval Devices." *American Journal of Nursing* (November): 2004–20.

Damanski, M. 1968. "Vesicoureteral Reflux in Paraplegia." *British Journal of Urology* 52: 168–72.

D'Ambrosia, R.D., ed. 1977. *Musculoskeletal Disorders*. Philadelphia: J.B. Lippincott.

Davis, Ross. 1975. "Spasticity Following Spinal Cord Injury." *Clinical Orthopedics and Related Research* 112: 66–75.

Downey, John, and Robert Darling. 1971. *Physiological Basis of Rehabilitation Medicine*. Toronto: W.B. Saunders. Pp. 3–136.

Dinsdale, S.M., et al. 1971. "Critical Psycho-Social Variables Affecting Outcome in a Regional Spinal Cord Centre." Pp. 193–96 in *Proceedings of the 18th Annual Clinical Paraplegia Conference*.

Dykes, Michael. 1975. "Evaluation of Muscle Relaxant: Dantrolene Sodium (Dantrium)." *Journal of the American Medical Association* 231, no. 8: 862–64.

Easterby, M. 1977. "Treatment for Pressure Sores and Statis." *Nursing Times*. April 14.

Edberg, E.L. 1973. "Prevention and Treatment of Pressure Sores." *Physical Therapy* 53 (March): 246–52.

El torai, I. 1977. "The Management of Pressure Sores." *Journal of Dermatology, Surgery and Oncology* 3 (October): 507–11.

Erickson, R.P. 1980. "Autonomic Hyperreflexia: Pathophysiology and Medical Management." *Archives of Physical Medicine and Rehabilitation* 61 (October): 431.

Falotico, J.B. 1979. "Pulmonary Emboli." *R.N.* (February): 47–500.

Fellows, G.J., and J.R. Silver. 1976. "Long-term Follow-up of Paraplegic Patients with Vesicoureteral Reflux." *Paraplegia* 14: 130–34.

Fitzmaurice, J.B., and A.A. Sasahara. 1974. "Current Concepts of Pulmonary Emboli: Implications for Nursing Practice." *Heart and Lung* 3, no. 2: 209–18.

Freehafer, A.A. 1966. "Para-Articular Ossification in Spinal Cord Injury." *Medical Services Journal of Canada* 12, no. 7: 471–78.

Freitag, J.J., and L.W. Miller. 1980. *Manual of Medical Therapeutics*. 23rd edition. Boston: Little, Brown.

Garfield, C.A. 1979. *Stress and Survival*. St. Louis: C.V. Mosby.

Glass, Alvin. 1974. "A Comparison of Dantrolene Sodium and Diazepam in the Treatment of Spasticity." *Paraplegia* 12: 170–74.

Glenner, G., et al. 1973. "Amyloidosis, Its Nature and Pathogenesis." *Seminars in Hematology* 1: 65–81.

Grant, Ragnar. 1964. "The Gamma-loop in the Mediation of Muscle Tone." *Clinical Pharmacology and Therapeutics* 5, no. 6: 837–47.

Gruis, M.L. 1976. "Assessment: Essential to Prevent Pressure Sores." *American Journal of Nursing* (November): 1762–64.

Gunther, M. 1976. "Emotional Aspects." In *Spinal Cord Injuries*, ed. D. Ruge. Springfield, Ill.: Charles C. Thomas.

Gutch, C.F., and Martha H. Stoner. 1971. *Review of Hemodialysis for Nurses and Dialysis Personnel*. St. Louis: C.V. Mosby.

Guthrie, R. 1969. "Surgical Management of Decubiti in Paraplegics." *Proceedings, 17th Veterans Administratio Spinal Cord Injury Conference*.

Guttman, Ludwig. 1963. "Observations on the Aetiology of Vesico-ureteric Reflux." *Paraplegia* 2: 184–185.

———. 1976. *Spinal Cord Injuries: Comprehensive Management and Research*. London and Boston: Blackwell Scientific Publications; Philadelphia: J.B. Lippincott. (1973, Oxford: Blackwell)

Guyton, Arthur. 1971. *Basic Human Physiology: Normal Function and Mechanism of Disease*. Philadelphia: W.B. Saunders.

———. 1981. *Textbook of Medical Physiology*. 6th edition. Philadelphia: W.B. Saunders. (1971, 4th edition.)

Hachen, H.J. 1974. "Anticoagulant Therapy in Patients with Spinal Cord Injury." *Paraplegia* 12: 176–87.

Hackler, R.H., et al. 1965. "Changing Concepts in the Presentation of Renal Function in the Paraplegic." *Journal of Urology* 94: 107–11.

Hardy, Alan G., and Reginald Elson. 1976. *Practical Management of Spinal Injuries*. New York: Churchill, Livingstone.

Hardy, A.G., and A.B. Rossier. 1975. *Spinal Cord Injuries: Orthopedic and Neurological Aspects*. Stuttgart: George Thiema Publications.

Harrison, J.H., R. Gittes, and A. Perlmutter, eds. 1979. *Campbell's Urology*. Vol. 2, 4th edition. Philadelphia: W.B. Saunders.

Harvey, A. McGehee, Richard J. Johns, et al. 1980. *Principles and Practices of Medicine*. New York: Appleton-Century-Crofts.

Heilborn, A. 1977/78. "Two Therapeutic Experiments on Stubborn Pain in Spinal Cord Lesions." *Paraplegia* 15: 368–72.

Hernandez, A.M., et al. 1978. "The Para-Articular Ossifications in Our Para-plegics and Tetraplegics: A Survey of 704 Patients." *Paraplegia* 16 (November): 272–75.

Hohmann, G.W. 1975. "Psychological Aspects of Treatment and Rehabilitation of the Spinal Cord Injured Person." *Clinical Orthopedics and Related Research* 112 (October): 81–88.

Horenstein, Simon. 1976. "Sexual Dysfunction in Neurological Disease." *Medical Aspects of Human Sexuality* (April): 7–13.

Howe, James. 1977. *Patient Care in Neurosurgery.* Boston: Little, Brown. Pp. 159–61.

Hume, M. 1976. "Examination of Venous Thromboembolism." *Hospital Medicine* (July): 56–65.

Hutch, J.A. 1952. "Vesico-ureteral Reflux in the Paraplegic: Cause and Correction." *Journal of Urology* 68: 457–67.

Isselbacher, K.J., ed. 1980. *Harrison's Principles of Internal Medicine.* 9th edition. New York, St. Louis, San Francisco: McGraw-Hill Blakiston.

Kahn, E. 1969. "Social Functioning of the Patient with Spinal Cord Injury." *Physical Therapy* 49 (July): 757–62.

Kaplan, Lawrence I. 1962. "Pain and Spasticity in Patients with Spinal Cord Dysfunction." *Journal of the American Medical Association* 182, no. 8: 918–25.

Kirilloff, Leslie H., and Ruth C. Maszkiewcz. 1979. "Guide to Respiratory Care in Critically Ill Adults." *American Journal of Nursing.* November.

Kollai, A.A. 1979. "Reciprocal and Non-reciprocal Action of the Vagal and Sympathetic Nervous System." *Journal of the Autonomic Nervous System* 1: 33.

Krupp, M.A., and M.J. Chattam. 1978. *Current Medical Diagnosis and Treatment.* Los Altos, Calif.: Lange Medical Publications.

Kyle, R.A., and E.D. Bayrd. 1975. "Amyloidosis: Review of 236 Cases." *Medicine* 54: 271–99.

Lance, James. 1974. "Mechanism of Spasticity." *Archives of Physical Medicine and Rehabilitation* 55, no. 2: 332–37.

Lane, Charles. 1964. "Introductory Remarks." *Clinical Pharmacology and Therapeutics* 2, no. 6: 803–4.

Lapides, J. 1974. "Neurogenic Bladder." *Urologic Clinics of North America* (February): 81–87.

Larrabee, J. 1977. "Physical Care During Early Recovery: The Person with a Spinal Cord Injury." *American Journal of Nursing.* August.

Leavitt, Lewis, and Beasley Wells. 1964. "Clinical Application of Quantitative Method." *Clinical Pharmacology and Therapeutics* 5, no. 6: 918–41.

Levy, N.B. 1974. *Living or Dying.* Springfield, Ill.: Charles C. Thomas.

Macrae, Isabel, and G. Henderson. 1975. "Sexuality and Irreversible Health Limitations." *Nursing Clinics of North America* 10, no. 3: 587–97.

Martin, Nancy. 1981. *Comprehensive Rehabilitation Nursing.* New York: McGraw-Hill.

McCormick, K. 1974. "Ventilating Failure Following Trauma." *Nursing Clinics of North America.* March.

McCutcher, R., ed. 1979. *Statistical Information Pertaining to Some of the Most Commonly Asked Questions About SCI.* Phoenix: National Spinal Cord Injury Data Research Center.

Merritt, John L. 1981. "Residual Urine Volume: Correlate of Urinary Tract Infections in Patients with Spinal Cord Injury." *Archives of Physical Medicine and Rehabilitation* 62: 558–61.

Miller, M.E., and M.L. Sachs. 1974. *About Bedsores*. London: Blackwell Scientific Publications.

Mirahmahdi, K.S., N.D. Vaziri, et al. 1982. "Survival on Maintenance Dialysis in Patients with Chronic Renal Failure Associated with Paraplegia and Quadriplegia." *Paraplegia* 20: 43–47.

Mirahmadi, K.S., and Robert L. Winer, et al. 1977. "Hemodialysis in Spinal Cord Injury Patients with Chronic Renal Failure." *Dialysis and Transplantation* 4: 6–10.

Montero, J., and D. Feldman. 1965. "Respiratory Problems of the Chronically Ill." *Archives of Physical Medicine and Rehabilitation* 46 (May).

Nepomuceno, Cecil, et al. 1979. "Pain in Patients with Spinal Cord Injury." *Archives of Physical Medicine and Rehabilitation* 60 (December): 605–8.

Nicholas, J.J. 1973. "Ectopic Bone Formation in Patients with Spinal Cord Injury." *Archives of Physical Medicine and Rehabilitation* 54 (August): 354–59.

Noback, C.R., and R.J. Demarest. 1981. *The Human Nervous System*. New York: McGraw-Hill.

Ott, R., and A. Rossier. 1971. "The Importance of Intermittent Catheterization in Bladder Re-education of Acute Traumatic Spinal Cord Lesions." Pp. 138–48 in *Proceedings of Veterans Administration Spinal Cord Conference*.

Papper, Saloman. 1971. *Clinical Nephrology*. Boston: Little, Brown.

Perkash, A., et al. 1979. "Experience with the Management of Thromboembolism in Patients with Spinal Cord Injury." *Paraplegia* 17: 322-31.

Petty, T. 1974. *Intensive and Rehabilitative Respiratory Care*. Philadelphia: Lea and Feberger.

Pearman, J.W., and E.J. England. 1973. *The Urological Management of the Patient Following Spinal Cord Injury*. Springfield, Ill.: Charles C. Thomas.

Pierce, D. 1971. *Dermatology in General Medicine: Decubitus Ulcers*. New York: McGraw-Hill.

Pierce, Donald, and V.H. Nickel. 1977. *The Total Care of Spinal Cord Injuries*. Boston: Little, Brown.

Pinel, C. 1976. "Pressure Sores." *Nursing Times*. February.

Price, S.A., and L.M. Wilson. 1978. *Pathophysiology*. New York: McGraw-Hill.

Rabin, Barry. 1980. *The Sensour Wheeler: Sexual Adjustment for the Spinal Cord Injured*. San Francisco: Multi Media Resource Center.

Rigoni, Herbert C. 1978. "Psychologic Coping of the Spinal Cord–Injured Patient." Downey, Calif.: Rancho Los Amigos Hospital (unpublished pamphlet).

Robbins, S.L., and R.S. Cotran. 1979. *Pathologic Basis of Disease*. Philadelphia: W.B. Saunders.

Roberts, Sharon L. 1976. *Behavioral Concepts and the Critically Ill Patient*. Englewood Cliffs, N.J.: Prentice-Hall.

Robmault, Isabel. 1978. *Sex, Society, and the Disabled: A Development Inquiry into Roles, Reactions, and Responsibilities*. New York: Harper & Row.

Rocha, Casas E., et al. 1976. "Prophylaxis of Venous Thrombosis and Pulmonary Emboli in Patients with Acute Traumatic Spinal Cord Injury." *Paraplegia* 14: 178–83.

Roddie, Ian C., F. William, and M. Wallace. 1975. *The Physiology of Disease*. London: Lloyd-Duke. Pp. 247–67.

Rothman, R., and F. Simeone. 1974. *The Spine*, Vol. 11. Philadelphia: W.B. Saunders.

Rubinow, A., and A.S. Cohen. 1978. "Skin Involvement in Generalized Amyloidosis." *Annals of Internal Medicine* 88: 781–85.

Ruge, D. 1969. *Spinal Cord Injuries.* Springfield, Ill.: Charles C. Thomas.

Rushworth, Geoffrey. 1964. "Some Aspects of the Pathophysiology of Spasticity and Rigidity." *Clinical Pharmacology and Therapeutics* 5, no. 6: 828–34.

Ryan, R. 1978. "Nursing the Patient with Thrombophlebitis." *Critical Care Update* (July): 21–32.

Sandowski, C. 1976. "Sexuality and the Paraplegic." *Rehabilitation Literature* 37: 322–37.

Scher, A.T. 1976. "The Incidence of Ectopic Bone Formation in Post-Traumatic Paraplegic Patients of Different Racial Groups." *Paraplegia* 14 (November): 202–6.

Scott, J.E.S. 1973. "An Experimental Investigation of Vesico-ureteral Reflux." *Paraplegia* 2: 181–82.

Small, M., H. Carrion, and J. Gordon. 1975. "Penile Prostheses: New Implants for Management of Impotence." *Urology* 5, no. 4: 479–86.

Smith, D.R. 1975. *General Urology.* Los Altos, Calif.: Lange Medical Publications.

Smithermann, C. 1981. *Nursing Actions for Health Promotion.* Philadelphia: F.A. Davis.

Spinal Cord Injured Hemodialysis Procedure Manual. 1976. Long Beach, Calif.: Veterans Administration Medical Center.

Stamey, T. 1980. *Pathogenesis and Treatment of Urinary Infection.* Baltimore: Williams & Wilkins.

Stanbury, J.B., et al. 1978. *The Metabolic Basis of Inherited Disease.* 4th edition. New York, St. Louis, San Francisco: McGraw-Hill.

Stefan, R., and B. Klaus. 1978. "Urinary Tract Infections." *Nurse Practioners* 3 (September-October): 33–38.

Stewart, T.D., and Alain B. Rossier. 1978. "Psychological Considerations in the Adjustment to Spinal Cord Injury." *Rehabilitation Literature* 39 (March): 75–80.

Stover, Samuel L., et al. 1976. "Disodium Etidronate in the Prevention of Heterotopic Ossification Following Spinal Cord Injury (Preliminary Report)." *Paraplegia* 14: 146–56.

Stryker, Ruth. 1972. *Rehabilitation Aspects of Acute and Chronic Nursing Care.* Toronto: W.B. Saunders.

Sutton, N. 1973. *Injuries of the Spinal Cord.* London: Butterworth.

Tarabulcy, E., P.A. Morales, and J.F. Sullivan. 1972. "Vesico-ureteric Reflux in Paraplegia: Results of Various Forms of Management." *Paraplegia* 10: 44–49.

Taylor, A.G. 1974. "Autonomic Dysreflexia in Spinal Cord Injuries." *Nursing Clinics of North America* 9: 4.

Tibone, James, et al. 1978. "Heterotopic Ossification Around the Hip in Spinal Cord–Injured Patients." *Journal of Bone and Joint Surgery* 60A (September): 769–75.

Travelbee, J. 1966. *Interpersonal Aspects of Nursing.* Philadelphia: F.A. Davis.

Travis, G. 1961. *Chronic Disease and Disability.* Los Angeles: University of California Press.

Tribe, C.R., and J.R. Silver. 1969. *Renal Failure in Paraplegia.* London: Pittman Medical Publishing.

Trieschmann, R. 1980. *Spinal Cord Injuries: Psychological, Social, and Vocational Adjustment.* New York: Pergamon Press.

Triger, D.R., and A.M. Joekes. 1973. "Renal Amyloidosis: A Fourteen-Year Follow-up." *Quarterly Journal of Medicine* (n.s.) 42: 15–40.

Turpie, A., and J. Hirsh. 1980. "Venous Thrombosis and Pulmonary Emboli: Guide to Detection and Prevention." *Hospital Medicine* (January): 22–47.

Vanderlinden, R.G., et al. 1974. "Electrophrenic Respiration in Quadriplegia." *The Canadian Nurse* 70: 23–26.

Van Hove, E. 1978. "Prevention of Thrombophlebitis in Spinal Injury Patients." *Paraplegia* 16: 332–35.

Van Rijswijk, M.H., and C.W.J. van Heusden. 1979. "The Potassium Permanganate Method." *American Journal of Pathology* 1: 43–54.

Vash, C. 1978. "Psychological Overview." In *Treatment of the Spinal Cord*, ed. M. Eisenberg. Springfield, Ill.: Charles C. Thomas.

Wade, J. 1977. *Respiratory Nursing Care, Physiology and Technique*. St. Paul: C.V. Mosby.

Watson, N. 1978. "Anticoagulant Therapy in the Prevention of Venous Thrombosis and Pulmonary Emboli in Spinal Cord Injury." *Paraplegia* 16: 655–69.

Weinstein, Sidney. 1962. "Phantoms in Paraplegia." Pp. 138–52 in *Proceedings, 11th Veterans Administration Spinal Cord Injury Conference*.

Weisenberg, Matisohu. 1979. "Pain and Pain Control." *Psychological Bulletin* 84: 1008–44.

Weiss, M. 1977. *Early Therapeutic Social and Vocational Problems in the Rehabilitation of Persons with Spinal Cord Injury*. New York: Plenum Press. Pp. 86–106.

Wharton, George W. 1975. "Heterotopic Ossification." *Clinical Orthopedics and Related Research* 112 (October): 142–49.

Wharton, George W., and T.H. Morgan. 1970. "Ankylosis in the Paralyzed Patient." *Journal of Bone and Joint Surgery* 52A (January): 105–12.

Wood, R., and K. Rose. 1978. "Penile Implants for Impotence." *American Journal of Nursing* 78, no. 2: 234–38.

Yashon, David. 1979. *Spinal Injury*. New York: Appleton-Century-Crofts.

Index